Current Topics in Microbiology 155 and Immunology

Editors

T-Cell Paradigms in Parasitic and Bacterial Infections

Edited by S. H. E. Kaufmann

With 24 Figures

Springer-Verlag
Berlin Heidelberg New York
London Paris Tokyo Hong Kong

Professor Dr. STEFAN H. E. KAUFMANN

Dept. of Medical Microbiology and Immunology,
University of Ulm
A.-Einstein-Allee 11, D-7900 Ulm

ISBN 3-540-51515-1 Springer-Verlag Berlin Heidelberg New York
ISBN 0-387-51515-1 Springer-Verlag New York Berlin Heidelberg

Library of Congress Catalog Card Number 15-12910
Printed in Germany

Phototypesetting by Thomson Press (India) Limited, New Delhi
Offsetprinting: Saladruck, Berlin; Bookbinding: B. Helm Berlin
2123/3020-543210 – Printed on acid-free paper.

Preface

It has been said that the development of vaccines against a variety of infectious diseases is among the greatest triumphs of immunology. Indeed, several pathogens have lost their horror through the availability of effective vaccination measures. Unfortunately, this does not hold true for the pathogens dealt within this volume. Malaria, schistosomiasis, leishmaniasis, leprosy, and tuberculosis together are prevalent in more than 100 countries, and over 400 million persons suffer from these diseases. It is becoming increasingly clear that the failure to control these infections in a satisfactory way is directly related to the complexity of their interactions with the immune system. These agents have lived with their hosts for long enough to give both—host and parasite—ample opportunity to develop a highly sophisticated interrelationship.

The central role of T lymphocytes both in acquired resistance to and pathogenesis of these microbes is well appreciated. In the beginning it may have been thought that acquired resistance against infectious agents is nothing but another aspect of the immune response, studied with soluble and particulate antigens. This simple concept has gradually changed, and it has become clear that the viability not only of the immune cells but also of the 'antigens' adds another dimension to the game. Several achievements in cellular immunology and molecular biology have now made it possible to better understand at least some mechanisms in this intricate interplay. It is my belief that the successful development of effective vaccines against diseases such as malaria, schistosomiasis, leishmaniasis, and leprosy will not be achieved before we thoroughly understand the complex relationships between host and predators. At the same time it appears that the study of such 'experiments of nature' can also provide information of general interest for the immunology community. It is the purpose of this volume to summarize in a paradigmatic way various T-cell mechanisms which contribute to resistance against and pathogenesis of these diseases. The topics include: (a) the wide array of effector mechanisms that are controlled by T cells; (b) the relative contribution of T_{H1} and T_{H2} lymphocytes to resistance and susceptibility; (c) the relevance of cytolytic T lymphocytes to protection; (d) the possible linkage of anti-infectious and autoimmune reactions by heat-shock proteins; (e) the in situ analysis of T-cell phenotypes and functions; and (f) the definition of T-cell epitopes and the design of recombinant carriers for vaccine development.

It is hoped that this collection is a fascinating one which is not only of interest for the scientist studying anti-infectious immunity but also of help for the pure immunologist. If so, it may aid in keeping immunology in close contact with reality.

Stefan H. E. Kaufmann
Ulm, Germany
August 1989

Contents

Schistosoma

Protozoa

Bacteria

Antigens and Carriers

List of Contributors

You will find their addresses at the beginning of the respective contribution

- Auriault, C.
- Bloom, B. R.
- Capron, A.
- Damonneville, M.
- De Vries, R. R. P.
- Goddeeris, B. M.
- Good, M. F.
- Gras-Masse, H.
- Jacobs Jr., W. R.
- James, S. L.
- Kaufmann, S. H. E.
- Koga, T.
- Lamb, J. R.
- Liew, F. W.
- Lugosi, L.
- Mehra, V.
- Miller, L. H.
- Modlin, R. L.
- Morrison, W. I.
- Munk, M. E.
- Ottenhoff, T. H. M.
- Pancre, V.
- Rothbard, J. B.
- Schoel, B.
- Scott, P.
- Sher, A.
- Snapper, S. B.
- Steinhoff, U.
- Tartar, A.
- Velge-Roussel, F.
- Wand-Württenberger, A.
- Wolowczuk, I.

Schistosoma

T-Cell Antigens and Epitopes in Schistosomiasis*

C. AURIAULT[1], I. WOLOWCZUK[1], M. DAMONNEVILLE[1], F. VELGE-ROUSSEL[1], V. PANCRÉ[1], H. GRAS-MASSE[2], A. TARTAR[2], and A. CAPRON[1]

1 Introduction

An ideal vaccine must duplicate the stimulus of natural infection and minimize the side effects that can interfere with its efficiency. New approaches to vaccine development using protein subunits or synthetic polypeptides must consider the problem of designing vaccines in such a way as to obtain optimal T-cell activity. Indeed, one characteristic feature of T-lymphocyte recognition is that foreign antigens are recognized by the T-cell receptor as peptidic fragments associated with class I or II major histocompatibility complex (MHC) proteins. Thus, knowledge of the T-cell repertoire in relation to the haplotype expressed is of primary importance in selecting, among the various mechanisms involved in the immune response, those leading to the more efficient protection against the infectious agents.

In recent years, immunological studies on parasitic models have clarified some of the components of the host-parasite interface, revealing it to be the result of a permanent and delicate balance between the parasite mechanisms of survival and the host factors of immunity. Although parasite models appear in many respects as relevant systems for the investigation of immunoregulatory mechanisms, the development of safe and protective vaccines against the major parasitic diseases has hitherto failed because of the complexity of the host-parasite relationships, an association that allows survival of both organisms. This is notably true in schistosomiasis, a metazoan infection that affects 200 million persons in the world, and that can be studied in various animal models (SMITHERS and TERRY 1965). *Schistosoma mansoni* infection is characterized by the presence of adult worms in the portal and mesenteric veins as the result of a complex migratory cycle initiated by cutaneous penetration of infective larvae (cercariae) living in water that transform into schistosomula under the skin of an appropriate host. The combined use of rodent models such as the mouse and the rat and of schistosomula in vitro culture during the past decade has made possible precise analysis of the immune

* The research described here was supported in large part by CNRS 624–Inserm U167; Financial assistance was also received from the UNDP/World Bank/WHO Special Programme For Research and Training in Tropical Diseases

[1] Centre d' Immunologie et de Biologie Parasitaire, Unité Mixte Inserm U167-CNRS 624, Institut Pasteur, 59019 Lille Cédex, France

[2] Laboratoire de Chimie des Biomolécules, Institut Pasteur, 59019 Lille Cédex, France

mechanisms in this infection. These laboratory models are usually described as "permissive" (mouse) or nonpermissive (rat) hosts according to their capacity to allow the parasite to reach sexual maturation and oviposition (CIOLI et al. 1977). In this chapter, we describe the role of T-cells in the immunity directed towards schistosomes in both permissive and nonpermissive rodent models. Several potentially vaccinating antigens have been characterized, and the molecular cloning of one of them, the P28 molecule (BALLOUL et al. 1987c), has allowed the determination of T-cell epitopes using synthetic peptides.

2 Components of the Immune Response to Schistosomiasis

Although eliciting the immune response to schistosomes in rat and mouse infections, the adult worm population seems relatively unaffected by immune effector mechanisms (concomitant immunity; SMITHERS and TERRY 1976). The protective immunity is directed against the larval pre- or post-lung stages and the involved humoral components, notably evidenced in the rat experimental infection (SMITHERS and TERRY 1965), whereas the mouse develops principally cellular-dependent protective mechanisms (SHER et al. 1975). Although cytotoxic T cells are not directly involved in killing mechanisms (BUTTERWORTH et al. 1979), much evidence has pointed to the preponderant role of T-lymphocytes in both rat and mouse antischistosome immunity, notably the strict thymic dependency of the essential components of the protective mechanisms developed against this parasite (CIOLI and DENNERT 1976; PHILLIPS et al. 1983). Indeed, T helper lymphocytes have the ability to act either by promoting B-cell proliferation and differentiation, thus allowing the production of specific antibodies of the adequate protective isotype in antibody-dependent cellular cytotoxicity (ADCC) or by directly activating effector cells in the absence of antibodies.

2.1 ADCC Mechanisms and Effector Cells

The rat model appears particularly valuable for the understanding of antibody-mediated immune mechanisms. Indeed, anti-μ treated animals, which cannot produce antibodies, failed to develop a high level of resistance to the infection normally observed in the controls, in which the worm population is almost entirely rejected 3–4 weeks after initial challenge, this rejection being itself followed by a strong and prolonged immunity to reinfection (BAZIN et al. 1980). This supports the view that rat resistance is in great part mediated by antibody-dependent mechanisms. In vitro culture and passive transfer of hyperimmune sera or monoclonal antibodies have allowed numerous studies of the effector mechanisms involving antischistosomula antibodies (CAPRON et al. 1982). These studies have demonstrated that ADCC appears as a potent mechanism in rat schistosomiasis and may also play a role in acquired immunity. Characteristic of ADCC mechanisms is that they do not involve conventional lymphoid cells but phagocytic cells such as macrophages (CAPRON et al. 1975), eosinophils (CAPRON et al. 1981), and blood platelets (JOSEPH et al. 1983), and that they imply a direct participation of anaphylactic isotypes in the cytotoxicity process. Indeed, a striking correlation is observed between the anaphylactic antibody response and the development of immunity to reinfection. IgG2a, the IgG anaphylactic subclass in the rat, is the first isotype able to mediate killing in eosinophil-dependent cytotoxicity. Later, IgE antibodies are involved in schistosomula killing in the presence of macrophages and platelets. The in vivo relevance of the key role played by these effector cells in protective immunity is evidenced by the fact that macrophages, eosinophils, and platelets from immune rats bear IgG2a (for eosinophils) or IgE (for macrophages, platelets, and eosinophils) on their membrane and are able to induce significant levels of protection after adoptive transfer to recipient rats (JOSEPH et al. 1983; CAPRON et al. 1984). The construction of rat-rat hybridomas and the production of monoclonal antibodies of various isotypes to *S. mansoni* have confirmed the protective activity of both IgG2a (GRZYCH et al. 1982) and IgE (VERWAERDE et al. 1987) in vitro in ADCC assays and in vivo.

2.2 Lymphokine-dependent Cytotoxicity

Regarding macrophages, a series of studies has pointed to the role of delayed-type hypersensitivity in the acquisition of protective immunity in the mouse (JAMES et al. 1983a). Indeed, intradermal injection of nonliving antigens with the bacterial adjuvant *Mycobacterium bovis* strain bacillus Calmette-Guérin (BCG) induces partial resistance to challenge infection in mice (JAMES and PEARCE 1988). This resistance is accompanied by an increase in lymphokine production and a macrophage activation.

Development of activated macrophages in the mouse infection correlates with the reduction in worm burden since manipulations known to activate macrophages induce partial resistance to schistosome infection, suggesting that these cells may play a major role in acquired immunity to this parasite in the mouse (JAMES et al. 1982).

Experiments involving nude mice indicate that T-cell function is critical for *S. mansoni* activation of macrophages, suggesting that in chronic schistosome infection the lymphokine-mediated pathway of macrophage activation plays a role similar to that currently observed in chronic bacterial infections. Indeed, when incubated with various schistosome antigens including living schistosomula (JAMES et al. 1983b), T-lymphocytes from *S. mansoni*-infected mice produced factors that are chemotactic/chemokinetic and activated macrophages for enhanced killing of the schistosome larvae. Moreover, macrophages recovered from the site of specific antigen challenge in immunized mice are activated to kill 3-h schistosomula in vitro. Furthermore, inbred mouse carrying known macrophage defects are not protected against challenge infection by primary infection in immunization with irradiated cercariae (JAMES et al. 1983, 1986).

A preponderant role seems to be played by the subpopulation of T cells bearing the L3T4 surface marker. The depletion of $L3T4^+$ cells in mice immunized once with irradiated cercariae reduced resistance when anti-L3T4 antibody was administered before the challenge infection such that depletion occurred during the time of skin penetration and dermal residence (Kelly and Colley 1988). These results suggest that a selective defect in T-cell functions, notably for production of macrophage-activating lymphokine(s) such as macrophage-activating factor (MAF), is manifested as a failure to produce activated larvicidal macrophages at the site of specific antigen challenge in vivo. Among the macrophage-activating factors, interferon-γ (IFN-γ) seems to play an important role, but other so far unknown factors are probably likewise involved. While most of the in vitro studies indicate that skin stage schistosomula are vulnerable to resistance mechanisms in immunized mice, other data show that for a brief period of time after leaving the lung, schistosomula become susceptible to attack by MAF-activated macrophages (Pearce and James 1986). Thus, schistosomula become rapidly resistant to antibody-dependent mechanisms, but the post-lung stage remains susceptible to the action of lymphokine-dependent macrophage effector functions, at least in the mouse model (Bout et al. 1981). Thus, several mechanisms of macrophage activation, depending on antibodies or lymphokines, can take place in the expression of macrophage cytotoxicity against the parasite.

As regards platelets, the demonstration of IgE-dependent functions of platelets in schistosomiasis (and filariasis) raised the question of their possible regulation by T-lymphocytes. Normal human platelets treated with culture supernatants from mitogen- or antigen-stimulated $CD4^+/CD8^-$ T cells developed the capacity to kill the larvae of *S. mansoni* in the absence of IgE antibodies. The physicochemical properties of the factors involved strongly suggested that IFN-γ was likely one of the lymphokine-stimulating platelet cytotoxicity. This hypothesis was confirmed by the fact that monoclonal and polyclonal anti-IFN-γ neutralized the induction of the platelet killer effect (Pancré et al. 1987). Moreover, the presence, at relevant concentrations, of IFN-γ in the supernatants of $CD4^+/CD8^-$ T-lymphocytes from *S. mansoni*-infected patients, and the direct inducer effect of recombinant IFN-γ clearly established that this lymphokine is a potent platelet activator, and that the interaction of platelets with IFN-γ leads to the production of schistosomicidal metabolites. The demonstration of interrelationship between IFN-γ and platelet function must be related to the work of Molinas et al. (1987), who have demonstrated that human IFN-γ is able to bind to high-affinity specific receptors on human platelets with an apparent equilibrium dissociation constant of $2 \times 10^{-10} M$.

The in vivo relevance of this effect was studied in the rat model. The passive transfer of normal rat platelets treated with rat recombinant IFN-γ to normal syngenic recipients on the day-of-challenge infection led to a high degree of protection (70%; V. Pancré et al., manuscript in preparation). In addition to its direct platelet cytotoxicity-inducing activity, IFN-γ acts on the IgE-dependent platelet cytotoxicity by enhancing the IgE receptor expression on the platelet membrane (Pancré et al. 1988).

A second inducing factor of platelet cytotoxicity, exhibiting a neutral pI has also been evidenced in $CD4^+/CD8^-$-stimulated T-lymphocyte supernatants. This factor was identified as tumor necrosis factor (TNF). Indeed, recombinant TNFβ and to a lesser extent TNFα induced normal platelets into cytotoxic effectors for *S. mansoni* schistosomula (DAMONNEVILLE et al. 1988). An additive effect of TNF and IFN-γ has also been observed. As described with IFN-γ, the in vivo relevance of the TNF-induced platelet-protective properties has been demonstrated by passive transfer of normal rat platelets treated with mouse TNFα (45%–65% protection; M. DAMONNEVILLE et al., manuscript in preparation).

As regards eosinophils, as mentioned above, both in man and rat model normal eosinophils can kill the larvae of *S. mansoni* in the presence of IgG and/or IgE antibodies. In the rat model, it has been shown that lymphocytes sensitized to *S. mansoni* antigens in vivo and challenged with the same antigen in vitro produce an activity that increases the killing potentiality of rat eosinophils in the presence of anaphylactic antibodies (VEITH et al. 1985). Moreover, a T-cell clone with the W3/13$^+$, W3/25$^+$ phenotype, characteristic of the rat T helper subset and specific for *S. mansoni* adult worm antigens, produced a similar activity. This eosinophil-enhancing activity was remarkably heat stable. The enhancement of several eosinophil functions by supernatants derived from stimulated or unstimulated lymphocytes from *Schistosoma haematobium* infected humans has been described, but this enhancing activity was not heat stable (SHER et al. 1983). The T-cell soluble factors seem to act not only by direct increase of the eosinophil-killing potentialities but also through their chemotactic capacities for eosinophils. These preliminary observations strongly suggest that several T-cell products act on eosinophil effector functions but, contrary to the case with macrophages and platelets, not by direct stimulation—rather, exclusively by enhancing antibody-dependent cytotoxicity. The participation of lymphocyte factors obtained after T-cell supernatant purifications or by recombinant DNA technology has been evidenced in hypodense eosinophil cytotoxicity assays in the presence of IgE. Enhancing effect was observed with interleukin 4 (IL-4), IL-5, HILDA, TNF-α, but not in the presence of IFN-γ (CAPRON et al. 1989). While the mode of action of these lymphokines must be determined, the findings obtained in the rat model suggest their effect not only on the release of helminthotoxic factors but also on the expression of surface receptor, notably the IgE receptor.

3 T-Cell Response After Immunization with Living Antigens

Vaccination with highly irradiated cercariae of *S. mansoni* induces partial resistance to subsequent infection in mice (MINARD et al. 1978). Several works have defined that in this model the protective immunity is T-cell dependent and is independent of lytic complement or tissue mast cell reactivity (SHER et al. 1982; JAMES and SHER 1983a). Mice of the inbred strains P/J or P/N (P) were found to develop minimal resistance to *S. mansoni* infection after exposures to irradiated cercariae, in contrast to other strains such as C57 BL/6 that showed strong vaccine-induced protection (JAMES and SHER 1983b). Extensive characterization of the immune responsiveness of the P mouse strain has demonstrated that the cell-mediated defect in this strain lies both in the ability of its macrophages to become activated and in the ability of its

T cells to produce the MAF, IFN-γ. It seems that resistance mechanisms induced by irradiated cercariae likewise involve humoral components under the control of T helper cells. Indeed, the role for protective humoral response has been suggested by studies in anti-μ suppressed mice (SHER et al. 1982) and by a report showing that sera from mice hyperimmunized by multiple exposure to irradiated cercariae can passively transfer resistance to naive recipients (MANGOLD and DEAN 1986). This suggests that resistance could involve several T-cell populations responsible for IFN-γ mediated activation of macrophages and protective antibody production. The ability of highly irradiated cercariae to induce substantial levels of immunity is therefore now well established. Little is at present known, however, about practical problems of technical feasibility, safety, and logistics of this type of vaccine, and this seriously hampers, its possible application to man.

4 T-Cell Response After Immunization with Nonliving Crude Antigenic Preparations

4.1 Induction of T-Cell Dependent Protective Immunity Using Crude Extracts of *S. mansoni* Adult Worms

Immunization against *S. mansoni* by intradermal injection of a soluble adult worm antigen preparation in combination with the bacterial adjuvant *M. bovis* strain BCG induced partial resistance to challenge infection in mice (JAMES 1985). In the C57BL/6 strain animals, the antibodies thus produced were predominantly directed toward a single antigen of 97 000 (Sm-97), present in cercariae, schistosomula, and adult worms and recently identified as paramyosin (PEARCE et al. 1986; LANAR et al. 1986). These studies have shown that resistance induced by the intradermal immunization of adult worm antigens in C57BL/6 mice was accompanied by sensitization for cell-mediated immune responses including delayed hypersensitivity. The level of resistance induced was influenced by the strain of BCG used, and isolated BCG cell wall did not reliably substitute for whole BCG organism as adjuvant. Despite the strong IgG response to Sm-97 paramyosin, no significant correlation between resistance to challenge infection and antibody level was observed. However, a strong correlation was noticed between resistance and antigen-specific cell-mediated reactivity, including IFN-γ production by T-lymphocytes in vitro and macrophage activation in vivo (JAMES and PEARCE 1988). This work suggests that in the mouse model, protection induced by nonliving soluble adult worm antigens is based on cell-mediated immune effector mechanisms.

The immunization of rats with an adult worm antigenic preparation was carried out to analyze the role of T cells in a model in which immune mechanisms require in great part the participation of thymus-dependent antibodies, especially antibodies of the anaphylactic subclasses. Thus, adult worm antigens (IPSm), specific T-cell clones derived from IPSm-primed lymph node cells, were prepared. Some clones (G5, E23), restimulated in an MHC-restricted manner and maintained in an IL-2 containing medium were demonstrated to exert in vitro and also in vivo helper activity (Pestel et al. 1985). Analysis of the surface phenotype of the IPSm-driven cell population revealed that the T cells expressed the markers W3/13 and W3/25 in agreement with the helper/inducer function of these cells. The in vivo helper activity was characterized by an accelerated production of IgG antibodies specific for 30- to 40-kDa schistosomula surface antigens and particularly towards the 38-kDa antigen. This surface antigen was demonstrated to be a major target present on the surface of living parasites (Dissous et al. 1981). Indeed, a rat monoclonal antibody of the IgG2a subclass precipitating only the 38-kDa component was shown to trigger in vitro schistosomula killing by eosinophils and passively to protect rats from infection by *S. mansoni* cercariae. Thus, it may be assumed that IPSm-specific T-cell clones could, at least in part, induce a protective immunity by favoring the production of antibodies of cytotoxic subclass directed towards the 30- to 40-kDa antigens.

4.2 Induction of T-Cell Dependent Protective Immunity Using Excretory/Secretory Products of *S. mansoni* Larvae

The schistosomulum antigens deserve particular attention since the larval stage appears to be the main target of the protective immune response to schistosomiasis in the rat model. A series of works have shown that the injection without adjuvant of schistosomula-released products (SRP-A) into rats (Auriault et al. 1984, 1985) induces a high cytotoxic IgE response. Up to 83% protection was observed when the rats were immunized with SRP-A before infection (Damonneville et al. 1986). The protective IgE response that developed after immunization was directed mainly towards an antigen of 26-kDa that was also recognized by the IgE antibodies of 35-day infected rat sera. The involvement of T-lymphocytes in the protective immune response elicited by the injection of SRP-A or of the 26-kDa molecule has been studied. SRP-A and purified 26-kDa antigen sensitized T-cell lines have been derived and tested (Damonneville et al. 1987) for their ability to produce in vitro IgE helper functions, IL-2 and MAF, or protective effect in vivo. The cells were maintained in culture in vitro by stimulation with schistosomulum homogenates. Interestingly, the SRP-A T cells were stimulated with antigenic preparations from different *S. mansoni* life-cycle forms, indicating the existence of common or cross-reactive epitopes recognized by the T-lymphocytes. Moreover, the SRP-A specific T-cell lines were shown to confer a significant protection to rat infected with *S. mansoni*. The sera of the rats passively transferred with SRP-A specific T cells displayed an important increase in the total IgE level whereas the total IgG level was not modified. These results corroborated those obtained by passive transfer experiments of anti-SRP-A IgE antibodies and confirmed that antigens secreted by the larvae are of particular interest notably in inducing a protective IgE production. The 26-kDa sensitized T-cells lines cocultured with spleen cells of SRP-A

Table 1. Functional analysis of 26-kD[a] specific T-cell clones after antigenic stimulation: IL-2, MAF production, and modulation of the IgE synthesis of the B hybrid B48-14 cell line

Cell clone supernatant		IL-2 activity[a]	MAF activity % of cytotoxicity[b]		IgE (ng/ml)[c]	Ratio
Control	Medium	906 ± 329	Medium	35.5 ± 1.0	Medium	1770 ± 417
	Positive	19 754 ± 2444	Normal rat serum	30.7 ± 3.4		
			Infected rat serum	57.5 ± 0.2		
			26-kDa specific T-cell line	58.0 ± 0.1		
6		2 985 ± 152		75.7 ± 4.3	2239 ± 29	1.26
11		4 309 ± 258		71.9 ± 13.3	1118 ± 222	0.63
21		1 028 ± 210		70.7 ± 12.2		
34		840 ± 208		80.4 ± 12.9	3821 ± 102	2.15
62		510 ± 420		40.2 ± 12.1	2401 ± 48	1.35
64		12 274 ± 2100		28.5 ± 20.4		
66		14 284 ± 1980		17.0 ± 10.3		
67		11 369 ± 2110		23.2 ± 11.7		

[a] IL-2 level was determined by [^{3}H]thymidine incorporation of concanavalin A stimulated lymphoblasts
[b] Percentage of dead larvae by peritoneal exudate macrophages incubated with T-cell supernatants
[c] Estimated by a specific competitive radioimmunoassay

immunized rats significantly enhanced IgE production in vitro. This strongly suggests that among the antigens present in the SRP-A, the 26-kDa molecule alone is able to induce T cells regulating the reaginic isotype production. Nevertheless, the use of unpurified splenic anti-SRP-A cells did not allow determination of whether the T-cell factor produced after antigenic stimulation acted directly on B cells or through other cell populations. It has been demonstrated that the secretion of IgE by a human myeloma cell line (U266) can be regulated by T-cell factors. Therefore, the rat B48-14 hybrid cell which produces a monoclonal IgE antibody specific for *S. mansoni* (Verwaerde et al. 1987) was used to test IgE synthesis regulation by the supernatants of 26-kDa antigen specific T-cell clones and hybrids. After antigenic stimulation, some of these cells liberated lymphokines able to modulate significantly the IgE synthesis produced by the B48-14 hybridoma cell line in vitro (Table 1). Besides their helper activity in cytotoxic antibody production, it may be assumed that the 26-kDa specific T-cell lines and clones exert a stimulating activity on the effector cells. To test this hypothesis, the cell supernatants were assessed for MAF production with a direct effect on the schistosomicidal activity of the activated macrophages. Among the 64 clones derived, six supernatants induced highly significant macrophage cytotoxicity towards the larvae in the absence of specific antibodies (Table 1).

The two clones 6 and 11 produced both IL-2 and MAF, the other five clones (21, 34, 64, 66, 67) produced either IL-2 or MAF. On the basis of these results, T-lymphocytes specific for the antigen released by the schistosomula or for the 26-kDa antigen alone have been shown to regulate the IgE response and presumably the effector functions of the macrophages. Knowledge of epitopes of the 26-kDa antigens generating T-lymphocyte activation is of primary importance in understanding the induction and the regulation of IgE production in schistosomiasis.

4.3 Induction of T-Cell Dependent Protective Immunity by the P28 Antigen of *S. mansoni*

1. The P28 antigen of *S. mansoni* has recently been shown to be a potential vaccinating molecule against schistosomiasis (BALLOUL et al. 1987a). Indeed, the native molecule, as well as the recombinant protein obtained after molecular cloning, was able to induce a strong protective immunity in the rat, mouse, hamster (BALLOUL et al. 1987b), and baboon (BALLOUL et al. 1987c). In the rat model, much work has been devoted to the antibody response and the protective effect of P28 antigen specific IgG and IgE antibodies in vitro in the presence of eosinophils as effector cells or in vivo after passive transfer to infected animals. The thymic dependency of the defense against *S. mansoni* led us to study the role of 28-kDa antigen specific T-lymphocytes in the protective effect observed in both rat and mouse models. Rat T cells, lines, and clones were prepared in a first step toward the purified native P28 antigen and examined for their helper and protective capacities (AURIAULT et al. 1987). The passive transfer of these cells to infected rats led to a significant protection (45%–85%), correlated with an increase in the production of 28-kDa antigen specific antibodies. This strongly suggests that epitopes of this antigen elicit T helper cells essential in stimulating prophylactic immunity, in which cytotoxic antibodies represent a major component. The stimulation of the native 28-kDa specific T cells with recombinant P28 demonstrated that the major T-cell epitopes were present and functional after molecular cloning. The identification of the major epitopes of the recombinant 28-kDa antigen has been undertaken using synthetic peptides deduced from the primary structure of the molecule. Three peptides comprising, respectively, amino acids 24–43, 115–131, and 140–153 were prepared according to their hydrophilicity, mobility, and accessibility profiles (Fig. 1). All three peptides were demonstrated to be B-cell epitopes in man as well as in the rat and the mouse models. Evidence for a 24–43 peptide-specific response of T-lymphocytes was determined by incubating nylon wool separated inguinal T-lymphocytes of infected (day 42) Fischer rats with several concentrations of 24–43 peptide either coupled to ovalbumin (OVA) or not (AURIAULT et al. 1988). The results demonstrated that 24–43 OVA induced a proliferative response whereas OVA alone did not (Fig. 2a). Moreover, inguinal T-lymphocyte blastogenesis from rat immunized with the recombinant P28 was estimated in the presence of 24–43, 140–153, and 115–131 peptides coupled or not to OVA. Peptides 24–43 OVA and 140–153 OVA induced a strong proliferative response whereas peptide 115–131 OVA did not (Fig. 2b). This suggested that peptides 24–43 and 140–153 contained a molecular structure recognized by the receptor of T-cell subsets specific for the P28 antigen. The necessary association of the peptide with a carrier raised the question of the presence of the functional agretope in the peptide sequence. The 24–43 and 140–153 peptides were homopolymerized (mean M_r 15 kDa) and used to test the lymphoblastic transformation of recombinant P28 antigen specific lymph node T-lymphocytes. These series of experiments showed that a slight proliferation of T cells was observed with the 24–43 peptide used at

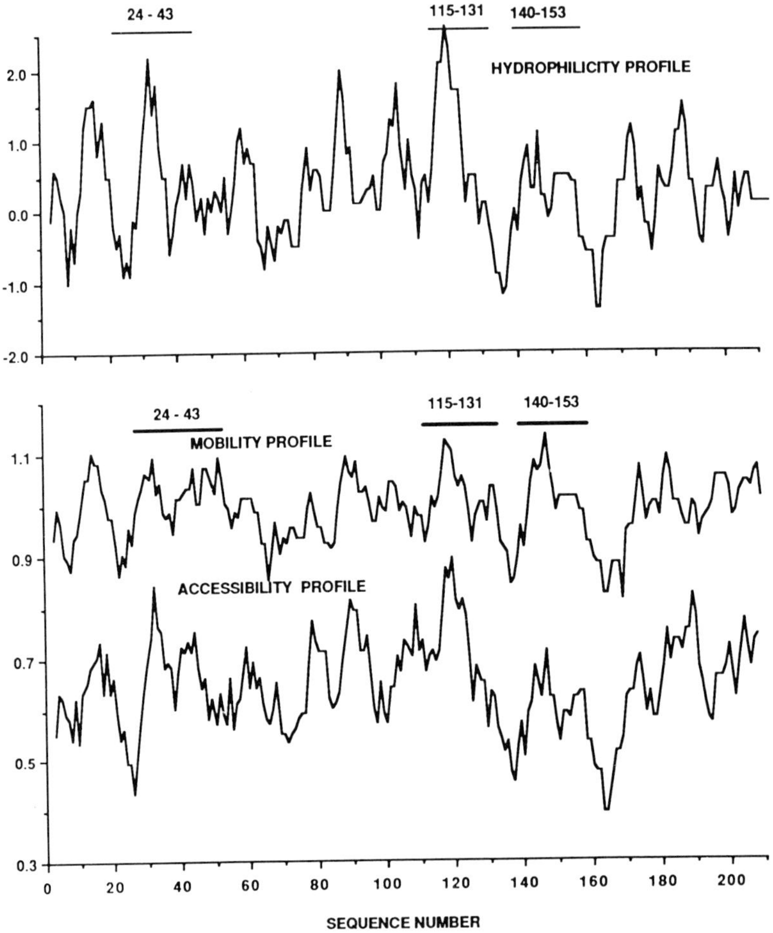

Fig. 1. Analysis of recombinant P28 antigen sequence according to mobility, hydrophilicity, and accessibility profiles

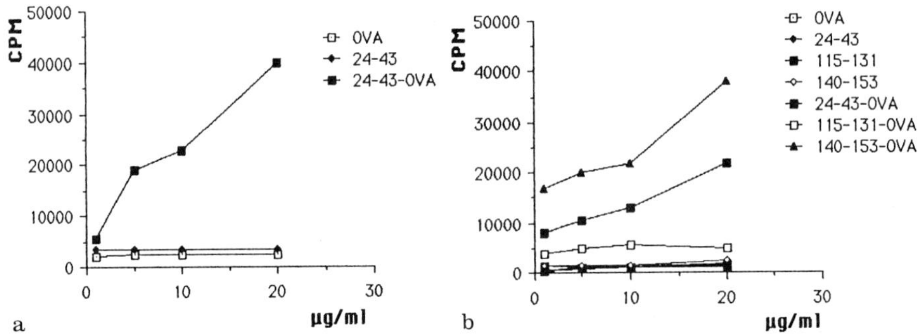

Fig. 2a, b. Proliferative response of T-lymphocytes from infected rats after stimulation with the 24–23 peptide coupled or not to OVA (**a**) and from rats immunized, with the recombinant P28 antigen after stimulation with the 24–23, 115–131, and 140–153 peptides coupled or not to OVA (**b**)

the concentration of 50 μg/ml, but that the stimulation was increased fourfold when the peptide was polymerized and reached the level of proliferation observed using the recombinant P28 as antigen. The proliferative response was not due to mitogenic effect of the polymerized 24–43 peptide since no response was observed with nonimmune T cells. In contrast, the 140–153 peptide homopolymerized or not did not induce T-cell activation. Taken together, these experiments demonstrate that even in the absence of carrier the 24–43 peptide was able to restimulate 28-kDa specific T-lymphocytes and suggest that this peptide probably contains at least one potent T-cell epitope. To determine the more precise location of this epitope the synthesis of peptides framing the amino (peptide 10–36) or the carboxyl (peptide 29–53) terminus of the 24–43 peptide were carried out. T cells from animals immunized with the recombinant P28 antigen were restimulated with the three peptides (10–36, 24–43, 29–53). The proliferation observed with the 10–36 peptide was higher than that observed with the two other peptides. Indeed, when the peptides were used at the concentration of 25 and 50 μg/ml, the proliferative response observed was twofold superior when the peptide 10–36 was used as antigen. In contrast, the stimulation induced by the two other peptides was similar, suggesting that probably two T-cell epitopes were located in the 24–43 peptide, one at the NH_2 terminus and the other at the carboxyl end.

T-cell lines specific for the 24–43 peptide were established by incubating nylon wool separated, 24–43 peptide primed inguinal T-lymphocytes with the 24–43 peptide coupled to OVA in a medium containing IL-2 for 1 month. After this period, the proliferation of the lymphoblasts in response to various antigenic preparations corresponding to several developmental stages of the parasite or the recombinant P28 molecules was tested (Table 2). Even after several weeks of culture, 24–43 peptide primed T-lymphocytes (exhibiting the W3/25 marker) were still stimulated with schistosome extracts. The maximum response was obtained with the adult worm antigen. Under the same conditions these cells exhibited a weaker but significant proliferative response when challenged in vitro with egg and schistosomula extracts. The stronger proliferative response was obtained when the recombinant P28 antigen was used as antigen whereas irrelevant antigens were unable to stimulate 24–43 peptide specific T-lymphocytes. The helper activity of 24–43 peptide specific T cells has been demonstrated after their passive transfer to rat immunized with the recombinant P28 antigen. Interestingly the helper effect concerns the P28 specific IgE production without modifying the production of IgG. Thus epitopes contained in the 24–43 peptide probably induce selectively T-cell populations involved in the production of IgE by means of the production of lymphokines (mainly IL-4 and, to lesser extent IL-5) known to regulate the synthesis of this isotype (Mosman et al. 1986; Coffman and Carty 1986).

2. Although the P28 antigen appeared to contain epitopes such as the 24–43 peptide, able to stimulate T cells to help the B-cell response, it was necessary to evaluate the T-cell epitopes implicated in antibody-independent cellular mechanisms also shown to be involved in the protection.

This study has been carried out with the mouse as model since, in contrast to

Table 2. In vitro proliferative response of 24–43 peptide primed Fischer rat inguinal lymph node cells cultured for 3 weeks in vitro and restimulated by various *S. mansoni* antigen preparations

Antigen source[a]	Concentration (μg/ml)	[^{3}H]Thymidine incorporation (cpm ± SD)	p[b]
Adult worms	5	11.241 ± 273	
	10	13.109 ± 705	
	20	15.006 ± 662	
	40	21.111 ± 943	< 0.005
Eggs	5	10.080 ± 766	
	10	10.160 ± 654	
	20	12.706 ± 463	
	40	17.864 ± 1162	< 0.05
Schistosomula	5	7.662 ± 422	
	10	8.913 ± 213	
	20	10.143 ± 702	
	40	13.701 ± 664	
Recombinant P28	5	40.112 ± 1472	
	10	46.260 ± 2024	
	20	52.413 ± 1962	< 0.005
OVA medium	20	450 ± 25	
		320 ± 32	

[a]Source of antigen added to IL-2 containing medium in the presence of syngeneic APC

[b]After 5 days of culture (16-h pulse, 0.5 μCi/well) results are expressed as the mean of two triplicate cultures. Student's *t* test was used for the comparison of means between nonstimulated cells and cells stimulated with 20 μg/ml schistosome extracts or 20 μg/ml of recombinant P28

the rat, T-cell dependent cellular immunity against schistosomes seems to play a preponderant role, as mentioned above. Moreover this model offers the possibility of estimating not only the repertoire of P28 antigen specific T cells involved in granuloma formation and consequently pathologic disorders but likewise the determination of immunodominant epitopes using P28 antigen high- and low-responder strains.

To determine whether recombinant P28 primed T cells can be activated by the native protein, lymph node T-lymphocytes of BALB/c mice immunized with the P28 antigen were monitored in in vitro proliferative assays towards various developmental stage antigens of *S. mansoni* (Wolowczuk et al., 1989). These specific T cells exhibited a dose-dependent proliferative response to adult worm and larval antigens, whereas a weak proliferation was observed with soluble egg antigens. Keeping in mind that the active immunization of recombinant P28 induced a strong protective immunity in the mouse, the involvement of humoral and cellular components in this protection was analyzed by passive transfer experiments. It appeared that (a) when infected mice were passively transferred with a L3T4$^+$-enriched P28 antigen T-lymphocyte population, a significant protection was observed (50% reduction in the worm burden), but (b) that no reduction in worm burden was observed when infected mice received recombinant P28 specific T-lymphocytes representing two T-cell subpopulations bearing L3T4$^+$ and Lyt2$^+$ phenotypes, in spite of a strong increase in the IgG response to

P28 antigen or to the 24–43, 115–131, and 140–153 peptides. In addition, a dramatic reduction in egg number in the liver of these animals was observed. Since the passive transfer of anti-P28 sera failed to protect mice against experimental infection, these results strongly suggest that, as expected in the mouse model, antibodies were not efficiently involved, and that the anti-P28 immunity depends on the interaction of L3T4^{+} T cells with effector cell populations. Indeed after in vitro stimulation with recombinant P28 antigen, P28 specific T cells were able to produce lymphokines inducing immune cells into cytotoxic effectors toward schistosomula. Supernatants of activated T cells were able to induce platelets and macrophages from normal BALB/c donors into killer cells. The implication of IFN-γ as one of these lymphokines was established with platelets but not with macrophages suggesting that the supernatants contained lymphokine(s) different from IFN and involved in this cytotoxicity (MAF, TNF).

Recombinant P28 specific murine T-lymphocytes exhibited a significant proliferative response after incubation with the peptides 24–43, 115–131, and 140–153 linked to OVA in the presence of antigen-presenting cells. The maximal response was obtained with the 24–43 peptide (Fig. 3a). The finest determination of the major T-cell site on the 24–43 peptide was undertaken using 10–36 and 29–53 peptides (Fig. 3b). As observed in the rat model, the major stimulation was obtained with the 10–36 peptide whereas the 29–53 peptide induced only a weaker proliferative response. These results suggest that one of the major T-cell epitopes of P28 antigen, in mouse and rat models, is located at the NH_2 extremity of the molecule.

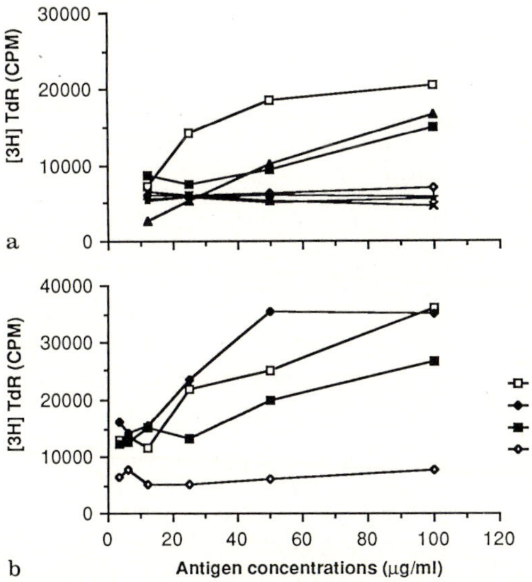

Fig. 3. **a** *In vitro* proliferative response of T-lymphocytes from mice immunized with the recombinant P28-1 antigen after stimulation with the 24–23, 115–131, and 140–153 peptides linked or not to a carrier protein (OVA). **b** Proliferative response of anti-rP28-1 T-lymphocytes using 24–23, 10–36, and 29–53 peptides coupled or not to OVA. After 5 days culture (16 h pulse, 0.5 μCi per well) results are expressed as the mean of two triplicate cultures. Student's *t* test was used for the comparison of means between non-stimulated cells and cells stimulated with peptides linked to a carrier protein. At the concentration 25 μg/ml and 50 μg/ml the proliferative responses were significantly different ($p < 0.05$)

Murine T cell lines that were 24–43 peptide primed were prepared, and the evidence for a schistosome-specific response of these cells was established by stimulating them with schistosome antigenic extracts of different developmental stages. A major stimulation was obtained with the adult worm antigens while the response observed with larval and egg antigens was weaker. The recombinant protein elicited a significant proliferation, as did the synthetic peptides framing 24–43 (10–36 and 29–53).

3. The genetic influence on the immune response in mice immunized with the recombinant P28 antigen has been studied (WOLOWCZUK et al., 1989). Various H-2 congenic strains of mice of BALB/c background were immunized with P28. Lymph node cell proliferation in response to P28 and its peptides was then analyzed (Fig. 4). As a first step of an immunogenetic approach, three strains were used: BALB/c (H-2^d), BALB/k (H-2^k), and BALB/b (H-2^b). It appeared clearly

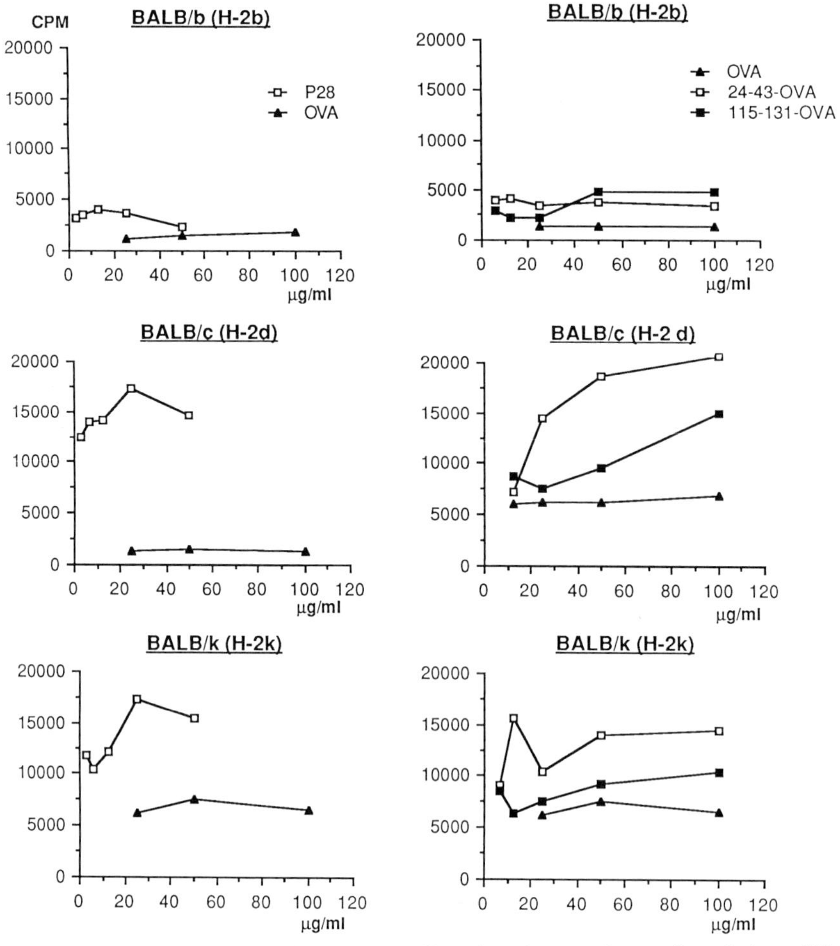

Fig. 4. Proliferative response of rP28-1 specific T-lymphocytes from mice of three different haplotypes on the BALB background with the rP28-1 antigen, the 24–23, and the 115–131 peptides linked or not on a carrier protein (OVA)

that d and k haplotype mouse T cells respond to the vaccinating protein P28 and the three peptides tested, while b haplotype expressing animals were low responders toward these antigens. These results were confirmed using mouse strains exhibiting these three different haplotypes ($H\text{-}2^{b,d,}$ and ^{k}) of another background (C57 Bl. 10). Although preliminary, these results suggest clearly that the genetic status of the individuals influence the immune response toward the P28 antigen. Taking into account the panmictic nature of the human population, a vaccination protocol with the P28 will have to consider both high and low responders to this antigen, and this will necessarily imply the construction of mimotopes sharing the same structure as the immunodominant epitopes but differing in physicochemical properties, allowing its recognition by the T-lymphocyte repertoire of low responders.

4. Analysis of the T-cell response toward P28 antigen and its peptides in rat and mouse infections has been carried out. The T-cell response was monitored on days 0, 7, 20, 35, 48, and 63 after *S. mansoni* infection. The results showed dynamic association of the T-lymphocyte populations able to be stimulated by the 24–43 and 115–131 peptides during the infection (I. WOLOWCZUK et al., in preparation). In the Fischer rat, a maximum response occurred against the 24–43 peptide as early as 8 days after cercariae infection, while at the same point the T-cell response towards the 115–131 peptides was very low but increased with the time of infection. Indeed, on day 63, the 24–43 and 115–131 peptides induced equivalent poliferative responses when used as antigens. Thus, this suggests that T-cell clones specific for the 24–43 epitope(s) could be present and numerous in the repertoire before the infection and thus stimulated early after cercariae infestation while other populations specific for the 115–131 epitope—less numerous—were educated and proliferated progressively during the infection. Moreover, it can be speculated that in *S. mansoni* infection the stimulation of T-cell clones expressing the 28-kDa antigen T-cell repertoire could depend on the different manners of antigen processing and presentation to these T cells in relation to the complex relationships between the parasite and its host. The purpose of future work will consist in delineating the functionality of each T-cell population according to these specificities. In the BALB/c mouse model contrary to the rat model, the response toward the two peptides was concomitant and decreased strongly after 63 days infection despite the presence of granuloma that excrete egg antigens, suggesting that the lymph node T-lymphocytes specific for the 24–43 and 115–131 peptide epitopes were not involved in the inflammatory reaction leading to the granuloma formation.

5 Concluding Remarks

This review has pointed out the important role played by T helper cells in *S. mansoni* infection and described the first analysis of the T-cell repertoire towards the P28 antigen that is a potential vaccinating molecule against this parasitic disease. If any conclusion can be drawn from this brief and in exhaustive survey, one would at least admit that a vaccine against schistosomiasis no longer represents an impossible dream. The study and the cloning of other vaccinating molecules, notably the 26-kDa antigen described above, are presently underway. It appears that according to the model studied, immunity toward schistosome could involve both antibody-dependent and -independent mechanisms, probably under the control of T_{H2} cells (producing IL-4 and IL-5) for the first and T_{H1} cells (producing IL-2, IFN-γ, TNF, and MAF) for the second (MOSMAN et al. 1986). The selective activation of T_{H1} and T_{H2} cells according to the immunogenetic status of the individuals in relation to the inducing epitopes appears henceforth of first priority. The use of synthetic immunogens cannot be discarded, at least to orient the immune response toward efficient immune component induction before or after immunization with the whole recombinant immunogens. It is obvious that the variety of responses induced by the immunogenic epitopes, together with the existence of a complex network of parasite escape mechanisms, must however moderate any excessive optimism. This points to the important role of the route and protocol of immunization and the nature of the adjuvant(s) used to optimize the vaccination. Research on the basic immunology of schistosomiasis has nevertheless allowed a clear understanding of the mechanisms of resistance and has also provided novel and important insights into the immune response and its regulation.

Acknowledgements. The authors would like to thank Claudine Colson and Marie-France Massard for secretarial expertise.

References

Auriault C, Damonneville M, Verwaerde C, Pierce RJ, Joseph M, Capron M, Capron A (1984) Rat IgE directed against schistosomula released products is cytotoxic for *Schistosoma mansoni* schistosomula in vitro. Eur J Immunol 14: 132–138

Auriault C, Damonneville M, Joseph M, Capron M, Verwaerde C, Billaut P, Capron A (1985) Defined antigens secreted by the larve of schistosomes protect against schistosomiasis: induction of cytotoxic antibodies in the rat and the monkey. Eur J Immunol 15: 1168–1172

Auriault C, Balloul JM, Pierce RJ, Damonneville M, Sondermeyer P, Capron A (1987) Helper T cells induced by a purified 28-kilodalton antigen of *Schistosoma mansoni* protects rat against infection. Infect Immun 55: 1163–1169

Auriault C, Gras-Masse H, Wolowczuk I, Pierce RJ, Balloul JM, Neyrinck JL, Drobecq H, Tartar A, Capron A (1988) Analysis of T and B cell epitopes of the *Schistosoma mansoni* P28 antigen in the rat model by using synthetic peptides. J Immunol 141: 1687–1694

Balloul JM, Grzych JM, Pierce RJ, Capron A (1987a) A purified 28 000 dalton protein from *Schistosoma mansoni* worms protects rats and mice against experimental *S. mansoni*. J Immunol 138: 3448–3453

Balloul JM, Sondermeyer P, Dreyer D, Capron M, Grzych JM, Pierce RJ, Carvallo D, Lecocq JP, Capron A (1987b) Molecular cloning of a protective antigen against schistosomiasis. Nature 326: 149–155

Balloul JM, Boulanger D, Sondermeyer P, Dreyer P, Capron M, Grzych JM, Pierce RJ, Carvallo D, Lecocq JP, Capron A (1987c) Vaccination of baboons with a P28 antigen of *S. mansoni* expressed in *E. coli*. In: Molecular paradigms for eradicating helminthic parasites. Liss, New York, pp 77–84

Bazin H, Capron A, Capron M, Joseph M, Dessaint JP, Pauwels R (1980) Effect of neonatal injection of anti-μ antibodies on immunity to schistosomes. J Immunol 124: 2373–2377

Bout D, Joseph M, David JR, Capron A (1981) In vitro killing of *S. mansoni* schistosomula by lymphokine activated mouse macrophage. J Immunol 127: 1–7

Butterworth AB, Vadas MA, Martz E, Sher A (1979) Cytolytic T lymphocytes recognize alloantigen on schistosomula of *Schistosoma mansoni* but fail to induce damage. J Immunol 122: 1314–1360
Capron A, Dessaint JP, Capron M, Bazin H (1975) Specific IgE antibodies in immune adherence of normal macrophages to *S. mansoni* schistosomules. Nature 253: 474–476
Capron A, Dessaint JP, Capron M, Joseph M, Torpier G (1982) Effector mechanisms of immunity to schistosomes and their regulation. Immunol Rev 61: 41–66
Capron M, Bazin H, Joseph M, Capron A (1981) Evidence for IgE-dependent cytotoxicity by rat eosinophils. J Immunol 126: 1764–1770
Capron M, Nogueira-Queiroz JA, Papin JP, Capron A (1984) Interaction between eosinophils and antibodies: in vitro protective role against rat schistosomiasis. Cell Immunol 83: 60–72
Capron M, Leprevost C, Torpier C, Capron A (1989) The second receptor for IgE in eosinophil effector functions. Prog Allergy (in press)
Cioli D, Dennert G (1976) The course of *Schistosoma mansoni* infection in thymectomized rats. J Immunol 117: 59–65
Cioli D, Knopf PM, Senft AW (1977) Study of *Schistosoma mansoni* transferred into permissive and non-permissive hosts. Int J Parasitol 7: 293–297
Coffman RL, Carty J (1986) T cell activity that enhance polyclonal IgE production and its inhibition by interferon γ. J Immunol 136: 949–954
Damonneville M, Auriault C, Verwaerde C, Delanoye A, Pierce RJ, Capron A (1986) Protection against experimental *Schistosoma mansoni* schistosomiasis achieved by immunization with schistosomula released products antigens (SRP-A): role of IgE antibodies. Clin Exp Immunol 65: 244–252
Damonneville M, Velge F, Verwaerde C, Pestel J, Auriault C, Capron A (1987) Generation and functional analysis of T cell lines and clones specific for schistosomula released products (SRP-A). Clin Exp Immunol 69: 299–307
Damonneville M, Wietzerbin J, Pancré V, Joseph M, Delanoye A, Capron A, Auriault C (1988) Recombinant tumor necrosis factor mediate platelet cytotoxicity to *Schistosoma mansoni* larvae. J Immunol 140: 3962–3965
Dissous C, Dissous C, Capron A (1981) Isolation and characterization of surface antigens from *Schistosoma mansoni* schistosomula. Mol Biochem Parasitol 3: 125–131
Grzych JM, Capron M, Bazin H, Capron A (1982) In vitro and in vivo effector functions of rat IgG2a monoclonal anti-*S. mansoni* antibodies. J Immunol 129: 2739–2744
James SL (1985) Induction of protective immunity against *Schistosoma mansoni* by non-living vaccine is dependent on the method of antigen presentation. J Immunol 129: 2206–2211
James SL, Pearce EJ (1988) Influence of adjuvant on induction of protective immunity by a non-living vaccine against schistosomiasis. J Immunol 140: 2753–2759
James SL, Sher A (1983a) Influence of adjuvant on induction of protective immunity against *Schistosoma mansoni* infection in mice vaccinated with irradiated cercariae. IV. Analysis of the role of IgE antibodies and mast cells. J Immunol 131: 1460–1467
James SL, Sher A (1983b) Mechanisms of protective immunity against *Schistosoma mansoni* infection in mice vaccinated with irradiated cercariae. III. Identification of a mouse strain P/N that fails to respond to vaccination. Parasite Immunol 6: 319–329
James SL, Lazdin JK, Meltzer MS, Sher A (1982) Macrophages as effector cells of protective immunity in murine schistosomiasis. I. Activation of peritoneal macrophages during natural infection. Cell Immunol 67: 255–266
James SL, Lazdin JK, Hieny S, Natovitz (1983a) Macrophages as effector cells of protective immunity in murine schistosomiasis. VI. T cell-dependent mediated activation of macrophage in response to *Schistosoma mansoni* antigens. J Immunol 131: 1481–1488
James SL, Skamene E, Meltzer MS (1983b) Macrophages as effector cells of protective immunity in murine schistosomiasis. V. Variation in macrophage schistosomulacidal and tumoricidal activities among mouse strains and correlation with resistance to reinfection. J Immunol 131: 948–953
James SL, Dehlois LA, Al-Zamel F, Glaven J, Langhorne J (1986) Defective vaccine-induced resistance to *Schistosoma mansoni* in P strain mice. III. Specificity of the associated defect in cell-mediated immunity. J Immunol 137: 3959–3967
Joseph M, Auriault C, Capron A, Vorng H, Viens P (1983) A new function for platelets: IgE-dependent killing of schistosomes. Nature 303: 810–812
Kelly EAB, Colley DG (1988) In vivo effect of monoclonal anti-L_3T_4 antibody on immune responsiveness of mice infected with *Schistosoma mansoni*. Reduction of irradiated cercariae-induced resistance. J Immunol 140: 2737–2745
Lanar D, Pearce ES, James SL, Sher A (1986) Identification of paramyosin as schistosome antigen recognized by intradermally vaccinated mice. Science 234: 593–595
Mangold BL, Dean DA (1986) Passive transfer with serum and IgG antibodies of irradiated cercariae induced resistance against *Schistosoma mansoni* in mice. J Immunol 136: 2644–2650

Minard P, Dean DA, Jacobson RJ, Vannier WE, Murrel (1978) Immunization of mice with cobalt-60 irradiated *Schistosoma mansoni* larvae. Am J Trop Med Hyg 26: 76–86

Molinas FC, Wietzerbin J, Falcoff E (1987) Human platelets possess receptors for a lymphokine: demonstration of high specific receptors for Hu IFNγ. J Immunol 138: 802–806

Mosman TR, Cherwinski H, Bond MW, Giedlin MA, Coffman RL (1986) Two types of murine helper T cell clones: definition according to profiles of lymphokine activities and secreted proteins. J Immunol 136: 2348–2357

Pancré V, Joseph M, Mazingue C, Wietzerbin J, Capron A, Auriault C (1987) Induction of platelet cytotoxic functions by lymphokines: role of interferon γ. J Immunol 138: 4490–4495

Pancré V, Joseph M, Capron A, Wietzerbin J, Kusnierz JP, Vorng H, Auriault C (1988) Recombinant human interferon γ induces increased IgE receptor expression on human platelets. Eur J Immunol 18: 829–832

Pearce EJ, James SL (1986) Post lung-stage schistosomula of *Schistosoma mansoni* exhibit transient susceptibility to macrophage-mediated cytotoxicity in vitro that may relate to late phase killing in vivo. Parasite Immunol 8: 513–527

Pearce EJ, James SL, Dalton J, Barrall A, Ramos C, Strand M, Sher A (1986) Immunochemical characterization and purification of Sm-97 a *Schistosoma mansoni* antigen monospecifically recognized by antibodies from mice protectively immunized with a non-living antigen. J Immunol 137: 3593–3599

Pestel J, Dissous C, Dessaint JP, Louis J, Engers H, Capron A (1985) Specific *Schistosoma mansoni* rat T cell clones. I. Generation and functional analysis in vitro and in vivo. J Immunol 134: 4132–4139

Phillips SM, Bentley AG, Linette G, Doughty BL, Capron M (1983) The immunologic response of congenitally athymic rats to *Schistosoma mansoni* infection. J Immunol 131: 1466–1474

Sher A, Smithers SR, MacKenzie P (1975) Passive transfer of acquired resistance to *Schistosoma mansoni* in laboratory mice. Parasitology 70: 347–354

Sher A, Hieny S, James SL, Asofsky R (1982) Mechanisms of protective immunity against *Schistosoma mansoni* infection in mice vaccinated with irradiated cercariae. J Immunol 128: 1880–1886

Sher A, Wader A, Joffe M (1983) The enhancement of eosinophil function by lymphocyte supernatants. Clin Exp Immunol 51: 525–532

Smithers SR, Terry RJ (1965) The infection of laboratory hosts with cercariae of *Schistosoma mansoni* and the recovery of adult worms. Parasitology 55: 695–706

Smithers SR, Terry RJ (1976) The immunology of schistosomiasis. Adv Parasitol 14: 399–410

Veith M, Pestel J, Loiseau S, Capron M, Capron A (1985) Eosinophil activation by lymphokines and T Cell clone products in the rat. Eur J Immunol 15: 1244–1250

Verwaerde C, Joseph M, Capron M, Pierce RJ, Damonneville M, Velge F, Auriault C, Capron A (1987) Functional properties of a rat monoclonal IgE antibody specific for *Schistosoma mansoni*. J Immunol 138: 4441–4446

Wolowczuk I, Auriault C, Gras-Masse H, Vendeville C, Balloul JM, Tartar A, Capron A (1989) Protective immunity in mice vaccinated with the *Schistosoma mansoni* P28-1 antigen. J Immunol 142: 1342–1350.

Cell-Mediated Immune Response to Schistosomiasis*

S. L. JAMES and A. SHER

1 Introduction

Schistosomiasis is caused by infection with blood flukes of the genus *Schistosoma*, of which three species (*S. mansoni*, *S. hematobium*, and *S. japonicum*) are the principal causes of disease in man. Schistosomiasis is a major health problem in the developing world, with an estimated 200 million persons infected and 600 million living in endemic areas where they are at risk of infection of (BERGQUIST 1987). This helminth parasite is acquired by man or other mammalian hosts through contact with a larval form found in fresh water. Having penetrated the skin, the larvae migrate and mature into adult worms living in the veins of the intestinal or urinary tract. Paired male and female worms produce hundreds to thousands of eggs per day, which are either excreted or become trapped in the body tissues of the host. Schistosomiasis is primarily a chronic disease, the pathology of which is associated with reaction to these trapped eggs. However the estimated mortality rate of approximately 1% (BERGQUIST 1987) translates into hundreds of thousands of lives lost annually.

T-cell mediated immunity has been implicated in two major phases of immune response to schistosomes: (a) in the mechanism of protection against infection that is observed in animals immunized by prior exposure to parasite antigens and (b) in formation of the granulomatous reaction to parasite eggs that plays a role in the pathology associated with chronic infection. Thus, further definition of T-lymphocyte function in schistosomiasis could lead to development of vaccination methods to induce resistance to infection, as well as to enhanced understanding of the chronic disease process.

The field of cellular immunology has recently been revolutionized by the observation that cloned $CD4^+$ T-cells can be separated into at least two phenotypes on the basis of differential lymphokine production (COFFMAN et al. 1988). According to this definition, T_{H1} cells preferentially produce gamma interferon (IFN-γ). interleukin 2 (IL-2), and lymphotoxin and mediate delayed hypersensitivity,

* The ongoing research described here is supported in part by grants from the Edna McConnell Clark Foundation and the World Health Organization

Immunology and Cell Biology Section, Laboratory of Parasitic Diseases, National Institute of Allergy and Infectious Diseases, NIH, Bethesda, MD 20892, USA

Current Topics in Microbiology and Immunology, Vol. 155

whereas T_{H2} cells are unique in their production of IL-4 and IL-5. Each of these T-lymphocyte subsets also exhibits different helper cell capability for stimulating B-cell differentiation and production of different immunoglobulin isotypes (e.g., IgG2a for T_{H1}, IgE for T_{H2}). In this chapter, we review briefly the observations that have led to recognition of the central role played by T-lymphocytes in the two principal facets of immune response to schistosomiasis and discuss how these recent discoveries in the area of cellular immunology may be applied to further define T-cell reactivity to schistosome antigens.

2 T-Cell Mediated Immunity in Resistance

It has been known for some time that in experimental animals primary exposure to living parasites, either by primary infection or immunization with radiation-attenuated parasites, leads to partial resistance to challenge schistosome infection (reviewed by SMITHERS and DOENHOFF 1982). Epidemiologic studies also suggest the development of acquired resistance in man (BUTTERWORTH and HAGAN 1987). This resistance has been attributed to development of protective immune responses. In the mouse, resistance induced by irradiated cercariae is dependent on T- and B-lymphocyte function but independent of complement, IgM-, or IgE-mediated immediate hypersensitivity (SHER et al. 1982). In mice immunized by a single exposure to irradiated cercariae, resistance is dependent on the presence of $L3T4^+$ cells, although hyperimmune mice (multiply exposed to irradiated cercariae) demonstrate resistance after $L3T4^+$ cell depletion (KELLY and COLLEY 1988). While the IgG fraction of sera from hyperimmunized mice can transfer partial protection to naive recipients, the level of resistance is lower than that observed in the serum donors. Furthermore, successful transfer has not been effected with sera from singly immunized mice although these animals are as strongly resistant to challenge infection as multiply vaccinated mice (MANGOLD and DEAN 1986). Therefore, the mechanism of resistance in singly vaccinated mice appears to be dependent on $CD4^+$ T cells and to involve the interaction of antibody and an immune effector cell.

A good candidate for the role of effector cell is the lymphokine-activated macrophage. Murine peritoneal macrophages treated with IFN-γ kill skin-stage schistosomula, as well as older (2- to 3-weeks) larvae, in vitro by a nonoxidative mechanism (reviewed in JAMES 1986a). We have recently determined that human monocyte-derived macrophages are likewise able to kill schistosomula when cultured in the presence of IFN-γ and colony-stimulating factors (S.L. JAMES and J.K. LAZDINS, manuscript in preparation). Although it has been reported that IL-4 can activate macrophages for tumor cytotoxicity (CRAWFORD et al. 1987), others have failed to repeat this finding (STOUT and BOTTOMLY 1988). In our hands IL-4 does not stimulate larvacidal activity by murine pertioneal macrophages (S.L. JAMES and M.S. MELTZER, unpublished data), indicating that macrophage activation for schistosomula killing is a strictly T_{H1}-dependent phenomenon. When present in high numbers, IFN-γ activated macrophages can kill larvae directly, in a non-antibody-dependent manner, as is the case with tumor cell targets; however, at lower effector:target ratios their antilarval activity is enhanced by addition of antibodies that serve to target their cytotoxic effects toward the parasite (James 1986a). T-lymphocytes from mice immunized once with irradiated *S. mansoni* cercariae proliferate and produce IFN-γ upon stimulation with schistosome antigens in vitro, and activated macrophages can be recovered from the peritoneal cavities of these animals after intraperitoneal injection of specific antigen (James et al. 1984b). Moreover, macrophages have been observed to accumulate around larvae at the sites of attrition of challenge infection in immunized mice (Ward and McLaren 1988; Crabtree and Wilson 1986). Collectively, these observations suggest that activated macrophages are likely to serve as effector cells of protective immunity in the irradiated cercariae model of resistance to schistosomiasis.

The most direct evidence of a role for this cell-mediated immune mechanism in resistance was derived from genetic studies. Whereas most inbred strains of mice respond to vaccination with irradiated *S. mansoni* cercariae by developing moderate to high levels of protective immunity against challenge infection, one inbred strain (P/JN) consistently fails to become resistant as a result of vaccination (James and Sher 1983). Peak levels of IgG antibodies to schistosomulum surface antigens produced by immunized P mice are equivalent to those in high-responder strain mice, and no differences in isotype representation have been noted, suggesting that differences in antibody levels are not responsible for the lack of protective immunity in this strain (Correa-Oliveira et al. 1984). However, P mice exhibit several defects in cell-mediated immune response, including lack of delayed hypersensitivity reaction, production of reduced levels of IFN by antigen or mitogen-stimulated T-cells, and decreased macrophage responsiveness to lymphokine-activating signals. Irradiated cercariae-immunized P mice do not produce activated, larvacidal macrophages upon stimulation with schistosome antigens (James et al. 1984a). Further studies using genetic crosses between a highly responsive strain, C57BL/6, that becomes strongly resistant following immunization and the low-responder P strain showed that in segregating generations the defect in macrophage function was significantly associated with the defect in development of resistance (James et al. 1987). This correlation is consistent with a cause-and-effect relationship, suggesting that macrophage activation is a requisite component of protective immunity in the irradiated vaccine model.

It is of interest that T-lymphocytes from singly immunized mice are at least as efficient as those from multiply immunized animals at IFN-γ production, a function of T_{H1} cells, which may explain why little if any increase in resistance is achieved by multiple immunization. However, preliminary experiments indicate that splenocytes from hyperimmunized mice are more proficient at IL-5 production, suggesting that multiple exposure to irradiated cercariae stimulates T_{H2} clonal expansion. Preliminary results also indicate that both singly and multiply immunized mice recognize a large number of schistosomulum antigens when analyzed for proliferation by T-cell immunoblotting. However the pattern of antigen recognition for IFN-γ production appears to be somewhat more restricted, suggesting that some antigens may be preferentially stimulatory for T_{H1} cells (F. Al-Zamel et al., manuscript in preparation). Further analyses of T-cell reactivity in the irradiated cercariae model are underway in our laboratories, with the hope that they will lead to identification of protective T-cell immunogens.

On the basis of these observations, we designed a nonliving vaccine against *S. mansoni* to induce cell-mediated immunity and examined its ability to protect mice against challenge infection. The conceptual basis of the vaccine was taken from early experiments of GREENE and BENACERRAF (1980) showing that immunization by the intradermal (i.d.) route enhanced T cell-mediated response, whereas immunization via the intravenous (i.v.) route was suppressive. In initial experiments, which concentrated on development of an effective immunization strategy rather than definition of a protective antigen, a crude antigenic preparation consisting of dead schistosomula was utilized and bacillus Calmette-Guérin (BCG) was added as a T-cell adjuvant. As would be predicted if cell-mediated immune mechanisms were protective, i.d. vaccination resulted in high levels of resistance (up to 85%, average of approximately 50%), while i.v. immunization failed to protect mice against challenge *S. mansoni* infection (JAMES 1985; JAMES and DEBLOIS 1986). In fact, in this model i.v. immunization appears to predispose against cell-mediated response, since the resistance observed in mice that had been subjected to i.v. immunization prior to i.d. immunization was reduced by some 70% (down to nonsignificant levels) as compared to animals immunized once or twice via the i.d. route only. In contrast, animals immunized with antigen by the i.d. route prior to i.v. exposure remained significantly resistant to challenge infection, indicating that once the protective immune response is established it is not readily reversed (S.L. JAMES, unpublished data). These observations strongly suggest that choice of the optimal immunization protocol is as critical to development of an effective vaccine as identification of a protective immunogen.

Intradermal vaccination is accompanied by sensitization for delayed hypersensitivity response, T-cell proliferation and IFN-γ production, and macrophage activation, whereas these responses are absent in unprotected i.v. immunized animals (JAMES 1986b). Strong correlative evidence that these T-cell activities are involved in protection was provided by the observation that P strain mice, found to be defective in macrophage activation in this as well as the irradiated cercariae model (JAMES et al. 1988), also fail to become resistant to challenge infection as a result of i.d. vaccination (JAMES and DEBLOIS 1986). Further proof was obtained from experiments in T- and B-cell deficient animals (Fig. 1). Nude mice failed to become resistant to challenge infection as a result of i.d. immunization, whereas their heterozygous littermates developed strong protective immunity. In contrast, mice that had been rendered B-cell deficient by injection from birth with goat anti-mouse μ-chain antisera (μ-suppressed mice), which had no detectable circulating antibodies against either larval surface antigens or larval/adult worm soluble antigens, showed levels of resistance (mean of 61%) comparable to those in untreated positive control animals following i.d. vaccination (Fig. 1a). Moreover, resistance in this model could be transferred to naive recipients by spleen cells but not serum from i.d. immunized mice (Fig. 1b). In these experiments, the level of resistance transferred with purified T cells (depleted of B cells by plating on anti-Ig-coated dishes, $<5\%$ Ig^+ cells remaining by immunofluorescence) was approximately equivalent to the level transferred with whole spleen cells from i.d. vaccinated mice. Since under all

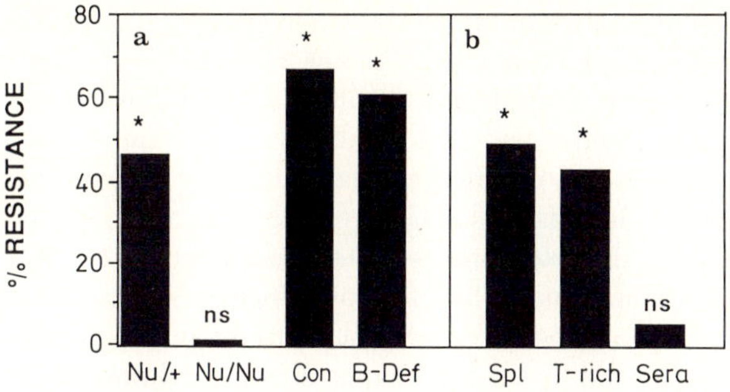

Fig. 1a, b. T-cell dependence of resistance to *S. mansoni* in the intradermal vaccine model. **a** Immunologically intact outbred Swiss nude heterozygotes (*Nu*/ +), T-cell deficient nude homozygotes (*Nu*/*Nu*), control C3H/HeN mice (*Con*), and B-cell deficient μ-suppressed C3H/HeN mice (*B-Def*) were immunized by i.d. injection with 1 mg protein of soluble adult worm antigens plus 5×10^6 colony-forming units of BCG. Four weeks later, they were challenged with 120 *S. mansoni* cercariae by percutaneous exposure of abdominal skin. After 6 weeks of infection, the adult worm burden was determined by portal perfusion. The percent resistance to challenge infection was calculated as [1 – (the number of worms present in the immunized groups divided by the number present in identical groups of mice that were given BCG alone)]. **b** C57B1/6J mice were irradiated (240 rad) and injected intraperitoneally with 1.5 $\times 10^8$ whole spleen cells from syngeneic mice immunized 4 weeks previously with 10^4 killed *S. mansoni* schistosomula plus BCG (*Spl*) or with 5×10^7 immune spleen cells that had been enriched for T-lymphocytes (*T-rich*) by two cycles of panning on anti-Ig coated plates ($< 5\%$ Ig^+ cells remaining). Alternatively, mice were injected i.v. with 0.5 ml of sera collected from similarly immunized animals. Either 5 days after cell transfer or 1 day after transfer of sera, mice were infected with 120 *S. mansoni* cercariae. Six weeks later, the animals were perfused and percent resistance was determined as described, based on comparison with the numbers of worms recovered from control groups that had received equivalent transfer of cells or sera from mice given BCG only. *Asterisks* refer to differences in challenge worm recoveries between experimental and control animal groups which were statistically significant at the $p < 0.05$ level

conditions of cell transfer thus far examined, helper activity for antibody production against soluble schistosome antigens was also enhanced in recipient animals, the experiments in B-cell deficient mice probably offer the most definitive proof of the cell-mediated basis of protective immunity in this model. While it is assumed that IFN-γ producing T_{H1} cells are responsible for resistance, this remains to be definitively proven in transfer studies using T-cell clones. Schistosome antigen-responsive T_{H1} (IFN-γ producing) and T_{H2} (IL-5 producing) clones have recently been generated in our laboratories, and these experiments are currently underway.

Having established a protective vaccination protocol using a crude nonliving schistosome antigen preparation, it remained to be determined whether a single protective antigen could be defined in this system, a condition that would make it more attractive as a potential human vaccine. It was initially determined that soluble schistosome antigens (either larval or adult worm) are at least as protective as membrane-containing fractions in this model (James et al. 1985). Because soluble antigens are more readily fractionated under the physiologic conditions required for testing cellular reactivity, identification of soluble T-cell immunogens was preferentially pursued. When soluble adult worm antigens were fractionated by gel filtration, the protective activity was observed to separate in a high molecular weight fraction that also contained immunogens for T-cell response (lymphokine production and elicitation of delayed hypersensitivity) as well Sm97, the major antigen recognized by sera from i.d. immunized mice (SHER et al. 1986; PEARCE et al. 1986).

Mice vaccinated i.d. with soluble schistosome antigens, although solidly resistant to infection, produce negligible levels of antibodies to larval surface antigens (JAMES et al. 1985). However, sera from these animals is reactive with soluble antigens, of which by far the most dominant is an internal antigen of M_r 97 000 (Sm97) (PEARCE et al. 1986). Gene cloning experiments led to the identification of this antigen as paramyosin, a myofibrillar protein that is a component of invertebrate muscle cells (LANAR et al. 1986). That antibody response alone to paramyosin is not sufficient for protection is demonstrated by the fact that sera from i.d. immunized, but nonresistant, P mice recognize this antigen (JAMES et al. 1988). However, in responsive mouse strains, vaccination with purified paramyosin sensitizes T-lymphocytes for proliferation and IFN-γ production (PEARCE et al. 1988), indicating that this serologically identified molecule is immunogenic for T_{H1} cells. Subsequent experiments have shown that purified paramyosin is protective in microgram quantities, when given i.d. in conjunction with BCG (PEARCE et al. 1988). Thus, one T-cell immunogen has already been identified in this model, and its vaccination potential will soon be evaluated in primates. However, soluble adult worm antigen preparations that have been depleted of paramyosin by affinity chromatography remain protective when administered i.d. with BCG, suggesting that other protective T-cell immunogens are also present in these antigenic mixtures (PEARCE et al. 1988). We are currently investigating their identity by T-cell immunoblotting techniques.

Thus, multiple observations point to a role for T-lymphocytes, and presumably T_{H1} cells in particular, in the mechanism of resistance to *S. mansoni*. Further research in this area could be of basic as well as applied interest, by identifying immunization techniques to preferentially stimulate one T-cell subclass over another and by defining the characteristics of antigens that are preferentially stimulatory for T_{H1} cells.

3 T-Cell Mediated Immune Responses in Pathogenesis

Mice chronically infected with *S. mansoni* develop many of the pathologic manifestations of schistosomiasis observed in man. These include eosinophilia, hepatosplenomegaly, hypergammaglobulinemia, and hypertension arising from blockage of portal venous circulation in the liver due to formation of cellular lesions (granulomas) and fibrosis around eggs trapped in these tissues (SMITHERS and DOENHOFF 1982). It has long been known that both the development of eosinophilia and granuloma formation are under T-cell control (WARREN et al. 1967; PHILLIPS et al. 1977). Moreover, T-cell clones from infected mice when stimulated with soluble egg antigens (SEA) produce soluble factors that augment the in vitro generation of egg granulomas and stimulate fibroblast proliferation (LAMMIE et al. 1986a).

Egg granuloma formation is a dynamic process whose regulation correlates directly with T-cell reactivity to SEA. Thus, peak granuloma formation and T-cell responsiveness occur during the early acute phase of infection, and both responses decline as the infection proceeds into the chronic phase. The latter phenomenon of down-regulation or modulation of granulomatous hypersensitivity appears itself to be a T-dependent process. In chronic *S. mansoni* infection suppression of granuloma formation can be adoptively transferred by a T-cell population whose activity can be depleted by either anti-$CD8^+$ treatment (previously interpreted as removing a suppressor-effector cell population) or anti-$CD4^+$ treatment (interpreted as depleting putative suppressor inducer cells), depending on the source of the donor cells and timing of the experiment. In *S. japonicum* infection both cellular and humoral (anti-idiotypic antibody) suppressor elements have been identified. Finally, a variety of egg antigen specific suppressor factors have been shown to be elaborated by T-cells from chronically infected mice. These factors appear to have anti-idiotypic activities which are postulated to be responsible for their modulation of T_H responses (PHILLIPS and LAMMIE 1986).

The hypothesis that granuloma formation is mediated by delayed-type hypersensitivity T-lymphocytes (T_{DH}) and modulated by classical suppressor T-cells must now be reexamined in the light of both the current debate concerning the existence of suppressor cells and the evidence for functional heterogeneity among T_H-lymphocytes. While it has been assumed that acute granuloma formation is the consequence of the action of T_{DH} cells, now classified as T_{H1} subset lymphocytes, the evidence is largely circumstantial. Thus, although SEA elicits a 24-h delayed-type footpad swelling response in mice at the acute stage of infection, an overlapping immediate response is also evident. Indeed, at the time of peak granuloma formation host T_{H2} responses such as eosinophilia, IgE, and IgG1 antibody production are also at peak or plateau levels (COLLEY 1981; SHER et al. 1977). Finally, recent studies in an in vitro egg granuloma model (LAMMIE et al. 1986b; B.L. DOUGHTY, personal communication) indicate that IFN-γ, the major T_{H1} derived macrophage-activating cytokine, actually suppresses granuloma formation rather than augmenting it when added to cultures. This observation is reminiscent of the inhibitory effect of IFN-γ that has been noted on T_{H2} cell activities (GAJEWSKI and FITCH 1988).

These considerations have led us to initiate a study of T_H subset regulation and cytokine function during granuloma formation. Initially, we have investigated the effects of antibody-mediated depletion of cytokines involved in T_{H1} versus T_{H2} responses on acute-stage granuloma formation and eosinophilia (A. SHER et al., manuscript in preparation). Repeated administration of an anti-IFN-γ monoclonal antibody, in a dose and regimen which in parallel experiments (P. SCOTT, personal communication) blocked healing of murine *Leishmania major* infection, failed to affect the size or cellular composition of granulomas in mice infected with *S. mansoni* for 8 weeks. Anti-IL-5 treatment, in contrast, had a pronounced but highly specific effect on the cellular response to schistosome infection. Acutely infected mice treated with a monoclonal antibody directed against this cytokine failed to develop peripheral blood or bone marrow eosinophilia and produced egg granulomas which were totally lacking in eosinophils. These lesions were slightly but significantly smaller than granulomas from untreated control mice, but were indistinguishable in terms of fibrosis and the presence of other inflammatory cell types. The above findings, in addition to establishing the IL-5 dependency of schistosome-induced eosinophilia, argue for the function of T_{H2}-associated cytokines within the granuloma and against a role for T_{H1} produced IFN-γ in the pathogenesis of the egg-induced tissue lesions. Preliminary data from direct measurements of T-cell cytokine activity support the conclusion that IL-5 responses to SEA predominate over IFN-γ responses during acute infection.

If then, as we propose, granuloma formation represents a primarily T_{H2} rather than T_{H1} response, the cellular basis of modulation of immunopathology must also be reexamined. Since IFN-γ is a down-regulator of in vitro granuloma activity (e.g., LAMMIE et al. 1986b) and is known to inhibit T_{H2} proliferation (GAJEWSKI and FITCH 1988), then production of this cytokine by either $CD4^+$ T_{H1} cells or $CD8^+$ lymphocytes themselves could account for granuloma modulation. Detailed functional studies on the T-cell subsets and cytokines involved in egg granuloma formation and regulation can now be designed to examine this issue directly.

4 Conclusions and Hypothesis: A Functional Dichotomy in the Role of T_H Subsets in Resistance and Pathology in Helminth Infections

The available evidence argues that during infection with schistosomes or other helminths T_{H2} responses predominate over T_{H1} responses, probably as a consequence of antigen presentation and dosage effects. Indeed, as we have speculated above, even the T cells responsible for schistosome granuloma formation which have been traditionally thought to be T_{DH} cells are likely to be predominately of the T_{H2} subset.

In contrast, the work on the schistosome vaccine models discussed here suggests that IFN-γ producing $CD4^+$ lymphocytes (T_{H1} cells) are important for resistance to infection. This conclusion is supported by recent data indicating that in vivo depletion with anti-IFN-γ but not anti-IL-5 significantly reduces the protective immunity induced by immunization with attenuated cercariae (A. SHER et al. manuscript in preparation) and by the finding that T cells from vaccinated mice, in contrast to those from infected animals, mount strong IFN-γ responses (JAMES et al. 1984 ; E.J. PEARCE, personal communication).

On the basis of the information currently available, we propose that in helminth infection the induction of T_{H2} activity represents a pathologic and *not* beneficially protective response against the parasite (Fig. 2). This concept is in direct contrast to theories proposing a protective role for T_{H2} associated IgE and eosinophil activities (e.g., CAPRON et al. 1987). Evidence for the latter hypotheses has emerged largely from studies in non-permissive hosts where the parasite may be more sensitive to the effects of these responses, and where the possible protective role of T_{H1} activities has not yet been adequately investigated.

If the natural response to chronic helminth infection is predominately T_{H2} dependent, it is logical that protective (e.g., vaccine-induced) immunity should involve a different and antagonistic T-cell function. As discussed above, IFN-γ is a

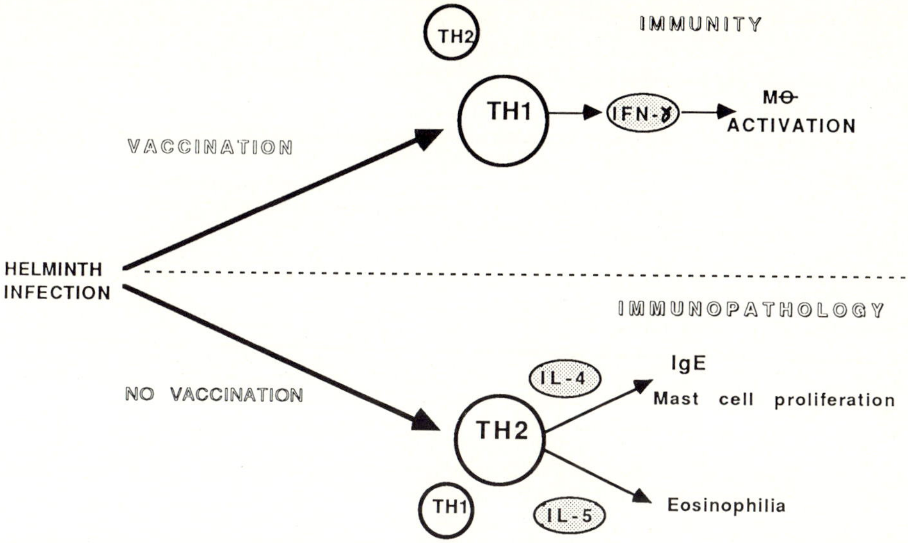

Fig. 2. A hypothesis concerning the roles of $T_H{}^1$ and $T_H{}^2$ subsets in immunity and immunopathology in schistosome and other helminth infections. As described in the text, we propose that helminth infections naturally stimulate $T_H{}^2$ responses which are associated both with parasite survival and immunopathology. In contrast, the induction of protective immunity results from the stimulation of the opposing $T_H{}^1$ subset leading to effector cell activation by IFN-γ

potent activator of macrophage effector cells, and the production of this cytokine by T_{H1} cells predominating in response to immunization could provide a parasite killing mechanism that is largely dormant during chronic natural infection. Thus, the selective induction of T_{H1} responses may represent a logical strategy for immunization and for improving the efficacy of exisiting antihelminth vaccines.

It is important to note that the functional dichotomy in T_{H1} and T_{H2} responses which we are proposing is in no way unique to helminth infections. In murine *L. major* infection T_{H1} cells have been shown to be protective whereas T_{H2} responses are associated with exacerbation (Scott et al. 1988; Heinzel et al. 1989). Indeed, recent data indicate that in situations in which T_{H2} responses are induced by this protozoan, both elevated IgE and eosinophilia—the noted hallmarks of helminth infection—are also induced (Heinzel et al. 1989; P. Scott, personal communication). Thus, the unusual immune responses elicited by worms may represent merely prominent T_{H2} activities which can be induced by other infectious or allergic stimuli under the appropriate immunoregulatory conditions.

Clarification of the dichotomy between T_{H1} and T_{H2} cell function in response to schistosome infection could allow definition of vaccination regimens to prejudice toward development of protective immune response. The knowledge gained by such studies should be helpful in the generation of immunization strategies against other infectious agents as well.

Acknowledgements. The authors wish to thank Drs. Philip Scott, Edward Pearce, Dan Colley, Bob Coffman, and Allen Cheever for helpful discussions and collaboration during various aspects of this work.

References

Bergquist R (1987) Schistosomiasis. In: Tropical disease research, a global partnership. Eighth programme report of the UNDP/World Bank/WHO special programme for research and training in tropical diseases. World Health Organization, Geneva

Butterworth AE, Hagan P (1987) Immunity in human schistosomiasis. Parasitol Today 3: 11–16

Capron A, Dessaint JP, Capron M, Ouma JH, Butterworth AE (1987) Immunity to schistosomes: progress toward vaccine. *Science* 23: 1065–1072

Coffman RL, Seymour B, Lebman D, Hirak D, Christiansen J, Shrader B, Cherwinski H, Savelkoul H, Finkelman F, Bond M, Mosmann T (1988) The role of helper T cell products in mouse B cell differentiation and isotype regulation. Immunol Rev 102: 5–28

Colley DG (1981) Immune responses and immunoregulation in experimental and clinical schistosomiasis. In: Mansfield JM (ed) The immunology of parasitic disease. Dekker, New York

Correa-Oliveira R, Sher A, James SL (1984) Defective vaccine-induced immunity to *Schistosoma mansoni* in P strain mice. I. Analysis of antibody responses. J Immunol 133: 1581–1586

Crabtree JE, Wilson RA (1986) The role of pulmonary cellular reactions in the resistance of vaccinated mice to *Schistosoma mansoni*. Parasite Immunol 8: 265–

Crawford F, Finbloom D, Ohara J, Paul W, Meltzer MS (1987) B cell stimulatory factor 1 (interleukin 4) activates macrophages for increased tumoricidal activity and expression of Ia antigens. J Immunol 139: 135–141

Gajewski TF, Fitch FW (1988) Anti-proliferative effect of IFN-gamma in immunoregulation. I. IFN-gamma inhibits the proliferation of $T_H{}^2$ but not $T_H{}^1$ murine helper T lymphocyte clones. J Immunol 140: 4245–4251

Greene MI, Benacerraf B (1980) Studies on hapten specific T cell immunity and suppression. Immunol Rev 50: 163–186

Heinzel FP, Sadick MD, Holaday BJ, Coffman RL, Locksley RM (1989) Reciprocal expression of interferon gamma or interleukin 4 during the resolution or progression of murine leishmaniasis. Evidence for expansion of distinct helper T cell subsets. J Exp Med 169: 59–72

James SL (1985) Induction of protective immunity against *Schistosoma mansoni* by a nonliving vaccine is dependent on the method of antigen presentation. J Immunol 134: 1956–1960

James SL (1986a) Activated macrophages as effector cells of protective immunity to schistosomiasis. Immunol Res 5: 139–148

James SL (1986b) Induction of protective immunity against *Schistosoma mansoni* by a nonliving vaccine. III. Correlation of resistance with induction of activated larvacidal macrophages. J Immunol 136: 3872–3877

James SL, DeBlois L (1986) Induction of protective immunity against *Schistosoma mansoni* by a nonliving vaccine. II. Response of mouse strains with selective immune defects. J Immunol 136: 3864–3871

James SL, Sher A (1983) Mechanisms of protective immunity against *Schistosoma mansoni* infection in mice vaccinated with irradiated cercariae. III. Identification of a mouse strain, P/N, that fails to respond to vaccination. Parasite Immunol 5: 567–575

James SL, Correa-Oliveira R, Leonard EJ (1984a) Defective vaccine-induced immunity to *Schistosoma mansoni* in P strain mice. II. Analysis of cellular responses. J Immunol 133: 1587–1593

James SL, Natovitz PC, Farrar WL, Leonard EJ (1984b) Macrophages as effector cells of protective immunity in murine schistosomiasis: macrophage activation in mice vaccinated with radiation-attenuated cercariae. Infect Immun 44: 569–575

James SL, Pearce EJ, Sher A (1985) Induction of protective immunity against *Schistosoma mansoni* by a nonliving vaccine. I. Partial characterization of antigens recognized by antibodies from mice immunized with soluble schistosome extracts. J Immunol 134: 3432–3438

James SL, Correa-Oliveira R, Sher A, Medvitz L, McCall RD (1987) Genetic association of defects in macrophage larvacidal activity and vaccine-induced resistance to *Schistosoma mansoni* in P strain mice. Infect Immun 55: 1884–1889

James SL, Salzman C, Pearce EJ (1988) Induction of protective immunity against *Schistosoma mansoni* by a nonliving vaccine. VI. Antigen recognition by nonresponder mouse strains. Parasite Immunol 10: 71–83

Kelly EA, Colley DG (1988) In vivo effects of monoclonal anti-L3T4 antibody on immune responsiveness of mice infected with *Schistosoma mansoni*. J Immunol 140: 2737–2745

Lammie PJ, Michael AI, Linette GP, Phillips SM (1986a) Production of a fibroblast-stimulating factor by *Schistosoma mansoni* antigen-reactive T cell clones. J Immunol 136: 1100–1106

Lammie PJ, Phillips SM, Linette GP, Michael AI, Bentley AG (1986b) In vitro granuloma formation using defined antigenic nidi. Ann N Y Acad Sci 465: 340–350

Lanar D, Pearce EJ, James SL, Sher A (1986) Identification of paramyosin as the schistosome antigen recognized by intradermally vaccinated mice. Science 234: 593–596

Mangold BL, Dean DA (1986) Passive transfer with serum and IgG antibodies of irradiated cercariae-induced resistance against *Schistosoma mansoni* in mice. J Immunol 136: 2644–2648

Pearce EJ, James SL, Dalton J, Barrall A, Ramos C, Strand M, Sher A (1986) Immunochemical characterization and purification of SM-97, a *Schistosoma mansoni* antigen monospecifically recognized by antibodies from mice protectively immunized with a nonliving vaccine. J Immunol 137: 3593–3600

Pearce EJ, James SL, Hieny S, Lanar D, Sher A (1988) Induction of protective immunity against *Schistosoma mansoni* by vaccination with schistosome paramyosin (Sm97), a non-surface parasite antigen. Proc Nat Acad Sci USA 85: 5678–5682

Phillips SM, Lammie PJ (1986) Immunopathology of granuloma formation and fibrosis in schistosomiasis. Parasitol Today 2: 296–302

Phillips SM, DiConza J, Gold J, Reid W (1977) Schistosomiasis in the congenitally athymic (nude) mouse. I. Thymic dependency of eosinophilia, granuloma formation and host morbidity. J Immunol 118: 594–599

Scott P, Natovitz P, Coffman R, Pearce EJ, Sher A (1988) Immunoregulation of cutaneous leishmaniasis: T cell lines which transfer protective immunity or exacerbation belong to different TH subsets and respond to distinct parasite antigens. J Exp Med 168: 1675–1684

Sher A, McIntyre S, von Lichtenberg F (1977) Kinetics and class specificity of hypergammaglobulinemia induced during murine infection. Exp Parasitol 41: 415–422

Sher A, Hieny S, James SL, Asofsky R (1982) Mechanisms of protective immunity against *Schistosoma mansoni* in mice vaccinated with irradiated cercariae. II. Analysis of immunity in hosts deficient in T lymphocytes, B lymphocytes and complement. J Immunol 128: 1880–1884

Sher A, Pearce EJ, Hieny S, James SL (1986) Induction of protective immunity against *Schistosoma mansoni* by a nonliving vaccine. IV. Fractionation and antigenic properties of a soluble adult worm immunoprophylactic activity. J Immunol 136: 3878–3883

Smithers SR, Doenhoff MJ (1982) Schistosomiasis. In: Immunology of parasitic diseases. Blackwell, Oxford

Stout R, Bottomly K (1988) Antigen-specific activation of effector macrophages by IFN-γ producing ($T_H{}^1$) T cell clones. J Immunol 142: 760–765

Ward R, McLaren DJ (1988) *Schistosoma mansoni:* evidence that eosinophils and/or macrophages contribute to skin phase challenge attrition in the vaccinated CBA/Ca mouse. Parasitology 96: 63–70

Warren KS, Domingo EO, Cowan R (1967) Granuloma formation around schistosome eggs as a manifestation of delayed hypersensitivity. Am J Pathol 51: 735–745

Protozoa

T-Cell Subsets and T-Cell Antigens in Protective Immunity Against Experimental Leishmaniasis

P. SCOTT

1 Introduction

Leishmaniasis is a chronic protozoal infection of man found in South and Central America, Mexico, Africa, Asia, and Europe. The parasite life cycle involves two forms, promastigotes and amastigotes. Promastigotes, found within the sandfly vector, initiate infection by invading macrophages. Once inside macrophages, promastigotes rapidly transform to the nonflagellated amastigote stage, which multiplies intracellularly. Eventually the infected cells rupture, and amastigotes reinvade other macrophages. The ensuing infection can manifest itself in a variety of ways, ranging from healing cutaneous lesions to non-healing cutaneous or visceral infections. This spectral nature is due, in part, to the host's immunologic response. Thus, although the various species of *Leishmania* exhibit significant differences, most species appear to be able to produce an inapparent, healing, or nonhealing infection. For example, although the visceral species of *Leishmania* have long been considered to produce a fatal infection in the absence of drug treatment, it is now known that these parasites may also produce relatively benign cutaneous lesions or completely inapparent infections (BADARO et al. 1986). Similarly, *L. braziliensis* species often produce a healing cutaneous lesion, although in a small percentage of patients severe mucocutaneous lesions develop.

There is a long history of active immunization of humans against cutaneous leishmanial infection (GREENBLATT 1980). Infection and subsequent healing is known to produce immunity in many cases, and, thus, controlled infections with low infecting doses at selected sites have been used to circumvent the development of disfiguring lesions. Although this form of immunization has been associated with a variety of complications, thus limiting its use, it demonstrates that immunization with an appropriate vaccine may be highly successful. Therefore, there presently is an effort to develop new vaccines for control of leishmanial infections.

The development of vaccines and the identification of protective immune effector mechanisms are strongly linked, and this has led to an effort to identify protective immunologic mechanisms in leishmaniasis. This chapter focuses on our current understanding of leishmanial immunity and how this understanding can be used to develop vaccines. An important aid in defining mechanisms of leishmanial

Department of Pathobiology, School of Veterinary Medicine, University of Pennsylvania, 3800 Spruce Street, Philadelphia, PA 19104, USA

Current Topics in Microbiology and Immunology, Vol. 155

immunity, as well as developing leishmanial vaccines, is the availability of several animal models of the disease, of which experimental leishmanial infections in mice have been the most studied. Similar to human infections, mice infected with *Leishmania* may develop either a healing or a nonhealing infection, which depends upon the strain and species of parasite, as well as the mouse strain. For example, C3H/HeN or C57BL/6 mice infected with *L. major* develop a cutaneous lesion at the site of inoculation that eventually heals, while BALB/c mice infected with the same parasite develop a progressive nonhealing infection that is ultimately fatal (Behin et al. 1979; Handman et al. 1979; Howard et al. 1980; DeTolla et al. 1981). Similarly, mice infected with *L. donovani* develop visceral infections, the extent of which is determined by the host's genetic makeup (Bradley and Kirkley 1977; Blackwell et al. 1980). It is from these animal models that our current understanding of leishmanial immunity is derived, and it is this knowledge that provides the framework for human studies and the design of effective vaccines.

2 Immune Effector Mechanisms in Leishmaniasis

2.1 Comparative Roles of Cellular and Humoral Responses

Self-cure and immunity to reinfection are generally attributed to cell-mediated immunity. Natural and experimental infections exhibit a strong association between healing and cellular responses. In addition, mice depleted of T cells by adult thymectomy, irradiation, and bone marrow reconstitution, as well as nude mice, are susceptible to infection (Preston et al. 1972; Mitchell et al. 1980). Most importantly, T cells transfer immunity, even in the absence of antibody (Rezai et al. 1980; Liew et al. 1982; Scott et al. 1986).

In contrast, there seems to be no protective role for antibodies in leishmaniasis during a natural healing infection. For example, increased antibodies are associated with chronic infections, while low antibodies are associated with healing infections, serum transfers fail to provide protection (Howard et al. 1984), and immune T cells transfer protection to B-cell deficient mice (Scott et al. 1986). Nevertheless, it is certainly possible that antibodies of the appropriate specificity might provide protection under the appropriate conditions, such as active immunization. In this regard, Handman and Hocking (1982) demonstrated that prior exposure of parasite to certain monoclonal antibodies led to increased killing by macrophages, and Anderson et al. (1983) demonstrated that parasites treated with another series of monoclonal antibodies produced significantly smaller lesions than controls.

2.2 Cellular Immune Effector Mechanisms

During both experimental and human leishmanial infections, T cells stimulated by antigen proliferate and produce lymphokines capable of activating macrophages. Since *Leishmania* are obligate intracellular parasites of macrophages, it is generally assumed that the main effector mechanism controlling parasite growth is lymphokine-mediated macrophage activation. In fact, a strong correlation between production of interferon-γ (IFN-γ) and resistance has been observed in cutaneous and visceral leishmaniasis (MURRAY et al. 1982; SADICK et al. 1986). In vitro, lymphokines such as IFN-γ can activate macrophages to kill *Leishmania* parasites (NACY et al. 1981; MURRAY et al. 1983). Moreover, the resistance of certain leishmanial strains to activated macrophage killing has been correlated with the ability of such strains to produce nonhealing infections in normally resistant mice (SCOTT and SHER 1986). Direct in vivo evidence that IFN-γ is important in controlling leishmanial infections comes from three types of experiments. First, it has been demonstrated that T cells producing IFN-γ can transfer resistance. These experiments have been performed both with T cells from protected animals (LIEW et al. 1985a) and with T-cell lines and clones (discussed further below). Second MURRAY et al. (1987) demonstrated that in vivo treatment of *L. donovani* mice with IFN-γ halted parasite growth. Third, recent in vivo depletion experiments with anti-IFN-γ monoclonal antibodies have proven that IFN-γ is a critical component in resistance to leishmaniasis. Thus, treatment of the normally resistant C3H/HeN mouse with anti-IFN-γ antibody led to the development of fatal *L. major* infections (BELOSEVIC et al. 1989; MULLER et al. 1989; P. SCOTT, unpublished data). The most straightforward interpretation of these results is that macrophages fail to be activated in the absence of IFN-γ. However, an additional factor contributing to susceptibility may involve stimulation of a different T-cell subset in the absence of IFN-γ, such as T_{H2} cells rather than T_{H1} cells (see below).

The fact that IFN-γ is the major effector molecule of the cellular immune response to leishmaniasis does not exclude the possibility that other mechanisms contribute to protection and resistance. For example, PANOSIAN et al. (1984) has described the presence of a T-cell population in healing mice that activate *Leishmania* infected macrophages by direct contact. The activity of these cells is not inhibited by cyclosporin A, and thus they do not appear to act by the secretion of IFN-γ (WYLER et al. 1987). Although the nature of these cells has yet to be determined, in the future they may provide a tool for defining potentially protective leishmanial antigens. Other cells that contribute to controlling visceral leishmaniasis are natural killer (NK) cells. NK deficient C57BL/6 bg/bg (beige) mice were found to be more susceptible to *L. donovani* than control mice, and this enhanced susceptibility could be overcome by transfer of cloned NK cells (KIRKPATRICK et al. 1985). These cells may contribute to resistance in a nonspecific way by producing IFN-γ or may act by an antibody-dependent cell cytotoxicity mechanism. If the latter were the case, then identification of the antigen specificities recognized by antibodies participating in this mechanism would be important. However, it should be noted that several attempts to demonstrate direct cytotoxic killing of infected macrophages have been unsuccessful (COUTINHO et al. 1984).

2.3 Role of $CD4^+$ and $CD8^+$ Cells in Protection

Both $CD4^+$ and $CD8^+$ cells might be involved in an effector mechanism relying on IFN-γ since both cell types are capable of producing IFN-γ (KAUFMANN 1988).

However, most experimental evidence suggests that $CD4^+$ T cells are the primary T-cell subset involved in leishmanial infection. Resistance to *L. major* infection can be transferred into nude mice with $Ly1^+$ cells, although the appropriate number of cells transferred is crucial in the outcome of the experiment (MITCHELL et al. 1981a). In addition, it has been demonstrated in a BALB/c vaccine model immunity can be transferred with $Ly1^+$ cells but not with $Ly2^+$ cells (LIEW 1987). Finally, TITUS et al. (1987) have shown that complete depletion of $CD4^+$ cells by in vivo treatment with anti-L3T4 monoclonal antibody leads to nonhealing infections in CBA mice. Nevertheless, there exists convincing evidence that $CD8^+$ cells may also contribute to healing, although possibly in a less dramatic way than $CD4^+$ cells. One of the most important observations in this regard came from studies which analyzed the ratio of $CD4^+$ and $CD8^+$ cells in the draining lymph nodes of resistant and susceptible mice. In BALB/c mice infected with *L. major* the majority of T cells capable of mediating delayed hypersensitivity were $CD4^+$, while in resistant animals an equal proportion were $CD4^+$ and $CD8^+$ (MILON et al. 1986). Moreover, 40% of the T cells infiltrating the leison site in resistant mice are $CD8^+$ cells (MCELRATH et al. 1987). In addition, depletion of $CD8^+$ cells by anti-$Ly2^+$ antibody treatment leads to delayed healing in CBA mice infected with *L. major* (TITUS et al. 1987). More dramatically, FARRELL et al. (1989) have demonstrated that anti-$Ly2^+$ treatment ablates the protective immunity that is elicited in BALB/c mice by intravenous immunization with irradiated promastigotes. In murine visceral leishmaniasis, depletion of either $CD4^+$ or $CD8^+$ cells inhibited protective immune responses, suggesting that both cell types are required for effective immunity (STERN et al. 1988). However, to date, both transfer of protection with $CD8^+$ cells alone and the ability to produce *Leishmania*-specific T-cell lines or clones with the $CD8^+$ phenotype have been unsuccessful.

2.4 Role of $CD4^+$ Subsets in Leishmaniasis

Some of the most important work to define the mechanisms responsible for the extreme susceptibility of BALB/c mice to *L. major* infection was done in the early 1980s by J. HOWARD and his colleagues. These investigators found that BALB/c susceptibility could be overcome by sublethally irradiating mice prior to challenge (HOWARD et al. 1981). Moreover, they demonstrated that this prophylactic effect could be reversed by transferring T cells from animals with progressive infection, or normal T cells, into the irradiated mice. However, T cells from animals that had been irradiated, infected, and had healed, transferred immunity. In both cases, the T cells mediating these effects were $Ly1^+$, $Ly2^-$ (LIEW 1987). The interpretation of these results was that BALB/c susceptibility was due to preferential stimulation of T suppressor cells following infection. The prophylactic effect of irradiation was not confined to BALB/c mice, but was also observed in other mouse strains infected with *L. major* as well as mice infected with *L. donovani* (HOWARD 1986; BLACKWELL and ULCZAK 1984). Even the P mouse, in which susceptibility was believed to be linked to a macrophage defect (NACY et al. 1983), was rendered resistant by irradiation, and as in the BALB/c model resistance was abrogated when normal T cells were

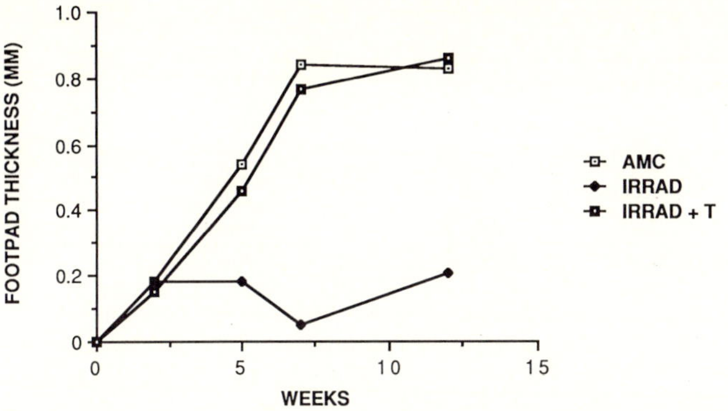

Fig. 1. Ability of irradiation to reverse the susceptibility of mice. P/J mice were irradiated with 550 rad and challenged in the footpad with $1 \times ^6$ *L. major* promastigotes, and the course of infection was monitored by following footpad swelling (*IRRAD*). One group of irradiated animals received 3.5×10^7 T cells prior to challenge (*IRRAD + T*). AMC, Age-matched controls. The mean lesion size of 5 mice per group is shown. The data presented is representative of two experiments

transferred into these mice (Fig. 1). These experiments conclusively established that T cells mediate both resistance and susceptibility to leishmaniasis. In addition, the data suggest that other suppressor mechanisms, such as nonspecific macrophage-mediated suppression (Scott and Farrell 1981), are secondary to a T-cell defect in susceptible animals. However, whether these T cells were actually acting as suppressor cells to decrease effector cell function remained controversial.

In 1985, Titus et al. found that partial elimination of $CD4^+$ cells by in vivo treatment with anti-L3T4 sera led to enhanced resistance in *L. major* infected BALB/c mice. This observation was followed up by the finding that the $CD4^+/CD8^+$ ratio differed dramatically in susceptible and resistant mice (discussed above). In addition, it was found that a *Leishmania*-specific $CD4^+$ T-cell line exhibiting the effector function of mediating delayed hypersensitivity, as well as producing macrophage-activating factors, transferred enhanced susceptibility to *L. major* infection (Titus et al. 1984). These observations led to the hypothesis that susceptibility in BALB/c mice was not due to suppression but rather was mediated by a heightened response to leishmanial antigens by $CD4^+$ T cells, leading to enhanced recruitment of macrophages to lesion sites, providing the necessary host cells for parasite growth. This hypothesis was supported by several additional observations. For example, it was found that susceptible mice exhibited enhanced myelopoiesis compared to resistant animals (Mirkovich et al. 1986), and that T-cell proliferation in the draining lymph nodes of BALB/c mice was significantly higher, at least during the early weeks of infection, than in the resistant C3H/HeN or C57BL/6 mice or even protectively immunized mice (Solbach et al. 1987; Heinzel et al. 1988; P. Scott, unpublished data; Table 1). Moreover, it was shown that newly recruited monocytes are relatively resistant to IFN-γ mediated macrophage activation and thus might well provide "safe targets" for leishmanial infection (Mirkovich et al. 1986; Hoover and Nacy 1984). Finally, experiments with nude mice appeared to confirm that large numbers of T cells might lead to exacerbation.

Table 1. Proliferation and lymphokine production by draining lymph node cells from BALB/c mice infected for 2 weeks with *L. major*

Cells	Proliferation		IL-2 (U/ml)	IFN-γ (ng/ml)	IL-4 (U/ml)	IL-5 (ng/ml)
	Bkg	Stimulated				
AMC	2998	35025	3.6	3.2	***5.2***	1.3
Fraction 1	8834	28340	2.8	2.9	***6.0***	***3.5***
Fraction 9	2552	10494	3.2	5.0	3.6	1.6

Lymphocytes were harvested from BALB/c mice 2 weeks after infection with *L. major*. Animals were immunized with Fraction 1 or Fraction 9 as previously described (SCOTT et al. 1987b) or were unimmunized (age-matched controls, AMC). Proliferative responses and lymphokine production was measured following stimulation with 50 μg/ml SLA. Lymphokine assays were performed as described in SCOTT et al. (1988a). Cells from uninfected animals failed to respond to SLA. Cells from animals immunized with only CP responded the same as AMC animals

Thus, while transfer of low numbers of Ly1$^+$ T cells could promote resistance to *L. major*, transfer of large numbers of Ly1$^+$ T cells led to susceptibility (MITCHELL et al. 1981a). Nevertheless, it was difficult to reconcile this hypothesis with the previous demonstration that T cells could in fact transfer immunity and with the rather clear-cut conclusions that different CD4$^+$ cell populations could mediate different outcomes in leishmanial infections (LIEW 1987).

It has long been postulated that CD4$^+$ T cells might consist of different subsets mediating different effector functions. This was confirmed in studies demonstrating that murine CD4$^+$ T-cell clones could be divided into two populations, designated T_{H1} and T_{H2} depending upon the lymphokines produced by the cells following mitogen or antigen stimulation (MOSMANN et al. 1986). T_{H1} clones produce exclusively interleukin 2 (IL-2) and IFN-γ while T_{H2} cells produce IL-4 and IL-5. Other lymphokines, such as IL-3 and granulocyte-macrophage colony-stimulating factor (GM-CSF) appear to be produced by both subsets, although in some cases quantitative differences exist. The evidence that differential stimulation of these two T-cell subsets explains susceptibility and resistance in leishmaniasis comes from two sets of experiments: an analysis of the lymphokines produced in susceptible and resistant mice and the demonstration that cells of these two phenotypes when transferred into normal mice have a dramatically different effect on infection. HEINZEL et al. (1989) characterized the lymphokine mRNA present in the draining lymph nodes of healing animals, both the genetically resistant C57BL/6 mouse and BALB/c mice rendered resistant by in vivo anti-L3T4 treatment, and the susceptible BALB/c mouse. Resistant mice contained high levels of mRNA for IFN-γ but little IL-4 message, while susceptible animals contained little IFN-γ mRNA but high levels of IL-4. That IL-4, a lymphokine controlling IgE responses, and IL-5, which is involved in eosinophil proliferation and differentiation, are produced during *L. major* infection in BALB/c mice, is suggested by the observation that these animals demonstrate high levels of circulating lgE and relatively high peritoneal eosinophilia following elicitation with leishmanial antigen (HEINZEL et al. 1989; P. SCOTT unpublished data). The evidence that these cells actually control leishmanial infection comes from the demonstration that T_{H1} cell lines transfer protection to *L. major* infection in BALB/c mice, while T_{H2} cell lines transfer enhanced susceptibility (SCOTT et al. 1988a; discussed further below).

The supposition derived from these findings is that susceptibility and resistance are directly related to the differential development of T_{H1} and T_{H2} cells. The interpretation of HOWARD's experiments within the context of this hypothesis is that irradiation prior to infection favors the development of T_{H1} cells, and that therefore these animals are capable of healing. However, if one transfers cells from infected BALB/c mice, which would be primarily of the T_{H2} phenotype, the prophylactic effect of irradiation is reversed. Transfer of normal BALB/c T cells, which have a bias in leishmaniasis toward T_{H2} development, would also lead to an uncontrolled infection. Similarly, partial depletion of $CD4^+$ cells by in vivo treatment with anti-L3T4 antisera would be analogous to irradiation, apparently primarily effecting T_{H2} development. Since our understanding of the factors controlling in vivo development of T_{H1} and T_{H2} cells is limited, it is difficult to determine how these immunologic manipulations alter the balance of $CD4^+$ T-cell subsets. However, it should be remembered that large numbers of $CD4^+$ cells promote susceptibility (and presumably T_{H2} development) in the BALB/c nude mouse, while low numbers of $CD4^+$ cells promote resistance (T_{H1} development; MITCHELL et al. 1981a). Since it would be expected that the proportion of a theoretical T_{H1} or T_{H2} precursor would be the same in the transferred populations, this experiment suggests that the actual number of $CD4^+$ cells stimulated may influence T_{H1} and T_{H2} development, at least in BALB/c mice.

The next important question is how these cells, and the lymphokines that they produce, control resistance and susceptibility in leishmaniasis. Since T_{H1} cells produce IFN-γ, a major macrophage-activating factor, it is not surprising that these cells mediate resistance. However, the role of T_{H2} cells and their lymphokines is less clear. At present, the best evidence suggests that these lymphokines act at the level of the macrophage, either by recruiting macrophages that are resistant to activation signals, down-modulating the ability of macrophages to respond to activating signals, and/or enhancing parasite growth within macrophages.

Enhanced in vivo production of the colony-stimulating factors IL-3 and GM-CSF has been correlated with susceptibility to leishmanial infection (MIRKOVICH et al. 1986; LELCHUK et al. 1988). In addition, high levels of colony-stimulating factors have been measured in cell lines capable of transferring enhanced susceptibility to leishmaniasis (RODRIGUES et al. 1987; SCOTT et al. 1988a; MULLER et al. 1989). Besides increasing the available pool of macrophages for parasites to infect, these lymphokines may also contribute to susceptibility by down-modulating IFN-γ mediated macrophage activation. Thus, when macrophages were treated with IL-3, IL-4, or GM-CSF prior to and during infection, no significant difference in parasite growth was observed. However, each of these lymphokines was found significantly to decrease the ability of IFN-γ to activate macrophages to kill or inhibit parasite growth (Fig. 2). That these in vitro observations may occur in vivo is suggested by the finding that macrophages specifically elicited with antigen in *L. major* infected BALB/c mice are relatively resistant to lymphokine-mediated activation (P. SCOTT, manuscript in preparation). In addition, although not observed in the experiment shown here, others have reported that IL-3 and GM-CSF augment parasite growth within macrophages (LOUIS et al. 1987; GREIL et al. 1988). Most importantly, the critical role of these lymphokines has been confirmed by in vivo experiments. It was

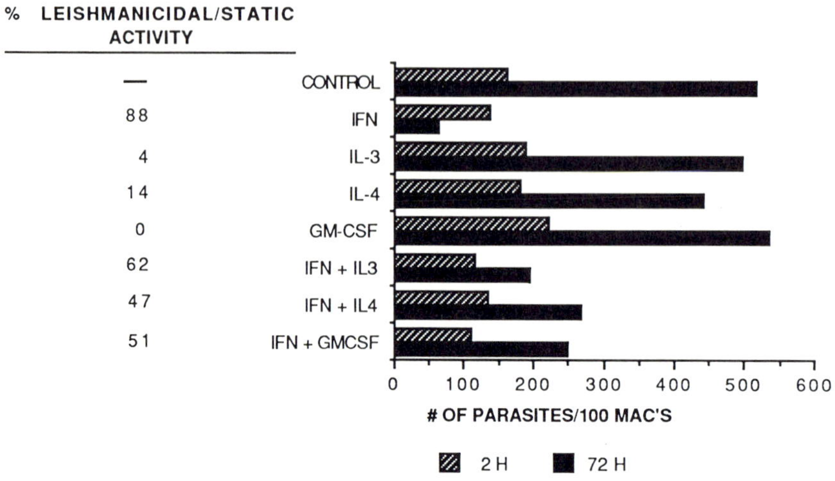

Fig. 2. Inhibition of IFN-mediated macrophage activation by IL-3, IL-4, and GM-CSF. BALB/c resident peritoneal macrophages were cultured in suspension at 36°C for 18 h with media alone or with the following recombinant molecules: IFN-γ (200 U/ml), IL-4 (300 U/ml), IL-3 (300 U/ml), and/or GM-CSF (300 U/ml). Macrophages were then infected with *L. major* amastigotes at a 2:1 ratio and allowed to incubate for 2 h. The macrophages were than washed, and the appropriate lymphokines were added for an additional 72 h (P. Scott, submitted for publication).

shown that in vivo administration of recombinant IL-3 and GM-CSF augments lesion development in both resistant and susceptible mice (Feng et al. 1988; Greil et al. 1988), while depletion of IL-4 using monoclonal antibodies enhanced resistance in BALB/c mice infected with *L. major* (Heinzel et al. 1989).

3 Experimental Vaccination

3.1 Vaccine Models

Although BALB/c is the mouse strain most susceptible to several cutaneous leishmanial species, it has been used extensively as a model for vaccine development. Mitchell et al. (1981b) found that BALB/c mice could be protected against fatal *L. major* infection by intraperitoneal immunization with frozen and thawed infected macrophages and the bacterial adjuvant *Corynebacterium parvum*. Irradiated or heat-killed promastigotes injected intravenously or intraperitoneally also provided excellent protecting against *L. major*, demonstrating that immunity could be obtained with either parasite stage (Howard et al. 1982). The ability to induce immunity by intravenous immunization with irradiated promastigotes was not confined to BALB/c mice. Other susceptible strains, such as P/J and SWR, and resistant strains, such as C3H/HeN and C57BL/6, could be protected against *L. major* infection (Howard 1986; P. Scott, unpublished data). In addition, protection

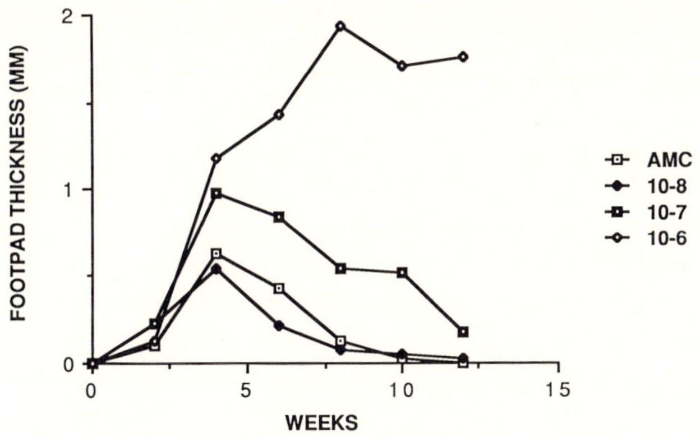

Fig. 3. Intradermal immunization in C3H/HeN mice. C3H/HeN mice were immunized intradermally with irradiated *L. major* promastigotes (150 krad). Three weeks later mice were challenged in the footpad with 5×10^5 *L. major* promastigotes, and the course of infection was monitored by following footpad swelling. The mean lesion size of 5 mice per group is shown. The data presented is representative of two experiments

against other leishmanial species has been shown (Howard et al. 1982; Alexander 1982). An important characteristic of this immunization with irradiated promastigotes was its route dependency. Thus, while animals were protected by intravenous or intraperitoneal immunization, subcutaneous immunization led to enhanced lesion development, and the enhanced susceptibility could be transferred with $Ly1^+$ T cells (Liew et al. 1985b). The necessity for systemic immunization with whole parasites is not confined to BALB/c mice. Thus, while normally resistant C3H/HeN mice immunized intraperitoneally with irradiated promastigotes demonstrate enhanced healing, mice immunized intradermally with low numbers of parasites develop significantly larger lesions than controls (Fig. 3). One interpretation of these results is that systemic immunization leads to preferential stimulation of T_{H1} cells, while subcutaneous immunization preferentially stimulates T_{H2} cells. The striking paradox here is that the intradermal route has traditionally been thought to favour cellular immunity, while the intravenous route favors stimulation of humoral immune responses (Greene and Benacerraf 1980). Most encouraging, however, are recent results suggesting that immunization with relatively defined antigens may overcome this route dependency (see below).

There are several approaches for defining what leishmanial antigens are responsible for inducing immunity. Since it has been difficult to define antigens recognized by T cells, antigens defined by their ability to be recognized by antibodies from infected or immunized animals have been tested for their ability to induce immunity One assumption made in these experiments is that the repertoire of antigens recognized by antibodies and T cells overlap. In addition, in some cases the molecules studied were demonstrated to have important biologic function. The first defined leishmanial antigen that demonstrated protective immunity in the BALB/c–*L. major* system was a glycolipid (now known as lipophosphoglycan, or LPG) derived from promastigotes (Handman and Mitchell 1985). This molecule is present on the surface of promastigotes and functions as a parasite receptor for macrophages (Handman and Goding 1985). LPG, purified using a monoclonal antibody that recognizes carbohydrate, induced significant protection against *L. major* in both BALB/c and C3H/He mice (Handman and Mitchell 1985). However, mice exhibited enhanced lesion development when the water soluble portion of the molecule, derived from the membrane-bound LPG, was used for induction of immunity (Mitchell and Handman 1986).

Another important promastigote surface antigen which has been tested for its ability to induce protective immunity is gp63. This molecule, isolated by Etges et al. (1985) and recently cloned by Button and McMaster et al. (1988), is a protease which also may contribute to promastigote attachment to macrophages (Russell and Wilhelm 1986; Chang and Chang 1986). When incorporated into liposomes and injected either subcutaneously or intraperitoneally, gp63 induced protection against *L. mexicana* in the relatively resistant CBA/Ca mouse strain; however, no significant protection was observed in BALB/c mice by gp63 given either subcutaneously or intraperitoneally (Russell and Alexander 1988). Other defined molecules that have been used for induction of immunity are less well characterized with regard to biologic function. For example, a membrane glycoprotein of molecular weight 46 kDa derived from *L. amazonensis* induced protection by both intravenous and subcutaneous immunization in CBA as well as BALB/c mice (Champsi and McMahon-Pratt 1988). One important conclusion from these experiments is that subcutaneous immunization can be successful with defined antigens. On the other hand, another *L. amazonensis* glycoconjugate, designated gp 10/20, enhanced lesion development (Rodrigues et al. 1987).

Another approach to isolation of protective leishmanial antigens is fractionation of a crude antigen preparation and identification of protective fractions. This approach was utilized to demonstrate that a soluble leishmanial antigen (SLA) preparation derived from promastigotes, when injected intraperitoneally with *C. parvum*, induced protective immunity against *L. major* infection in BALB/c mice equivalent to that obtained with whole promastigotes (Scott et al. 1987a). In addition, mice immunized subcutaneously with SLA and *C. parvum* also exhibited protection against infection, although not as complete as that obtained following intraperitoneal immunization (P. Scott, manuscript in preparation). Further fractionation of SLA by anion exchange liquid chromatography yielded two fractions recognized by T cells from SLA immunized mice, designated fractions 1 and 9. However, when used to immunize mice, only fraction 9 induced protection (Scott et al. 1987b). This antigen pool contains a negatively charged group of molecules, including both proteins and DNA. It was shown that proteins within the fraction are responsible for protection, and since the fraction contains less than 1% of the total protein in SLA and is immunogenic at one-tenth of the SLA concentration required for protection, it represents a significant purification of the protective molecules in SLA.

One question which these results raised was why fraction 1, which was recognized by T cells from protected mice, failed to induce protection. To determine whether fractions 1 and 9 stimulated different $CD4^+$ T cell subsets, lymphokines produced by cells obtained from the draining lymph nodes of 2-week infected mice were analyzed. It was found that lymphocytes from mice protectively immunized with fraction 9 produced elevated levels of IFN-γ, while cells from fraction 1 immunized mice produced more IL-4 and IL-5 (Table 1). These results suggest that T_{H1} cells are primed following exposure to fraction 9, while T_{H2} cells are primed by fraction 1. However, it should be noted that a contribution of $CD8^+$ cells in the production of IFN-γ is not excluded, since the experiments were performed with unfractionated cells. Nevertheless, the data serve to further support the hypothesis that resistance and susceptibility in murine leishmaniasis can be attributed to differential stimulation of $CD4^+$ T-cell subsets.

A similar approach to define protective antigens utilized sodium dodecyl sulfate polyacrylamide gel (SDS-PAGE) fractionation. Fractions of different molecular weights obtained by running an extract of whole promastigotes on an SDS-PAGE were electroeluted and used to immunize mice (FROMMEL et al. 1988). Antigens in the molecular weight ranges of less than 20 kDa, 20–30 kDa, and 67–94 kDa protected against *L. mexicana* infection in BALB/c mice. Although both of these approaches to parasite fractionation (anion exchange chromatography and SDS-PAGE) have provided semipurified antigens that protect, further identification of the protective antigens within these fractions may be relatively difficult. One method to facilitate the isolation of the protective immunogens within these fractions is identification of the antigens recognized by protective T cells.

3.2 Protective T-Cell Lines

The most direct way to define a protective immunogen in leishmaniasis is to identify the antigens recognized by protective T cells. Two advances have facilitated this approach. The first is the ability to make T-cell lines and clones, and the second is to identify the antigens recognized by these cells using T-cell immunoblotting. One of the first attempts to produce a protective T-cell line in leishmaniasis was unsuccessful. Thus, instead of transferring protection, the cells induced enhanced lesions (TITUS et al. 1984). Since these cells were obtained from animals that were subcutaneously immunized, which would not provide protective immunity, these results are not surprising. However, supernatants from these cells were shown to contain macrophage-activating activity inhibited by anti-IFN-γ treatment, suggesting that they belonged to the T_{H1} cell type (MULLER et al. 1989). One likely interpretation of these results is that not all T_{H1} cells will by definition be protective, and that antigen specificity is crucial in their function (MULLER et al. 1989). If this is the case, the importance of testing T-cell lines and clones in animal models for their protective capacity is paramount, since not all T cells producing IFN-γ would by definition be protective. However, a complete characterization of the lymphokines produced by this cell line is needed to ensure that it does not represent a mixed cell population.

Another cell line shown to exacerbate experimental leishmanial infections was obtained from mice immunized with the *L. mexicana* antigen gp10/20 (RODRIGUES et al. 1987). Although these cells have not been characterized as to $CD4^+$ subset, they have been shown to produce high levels of colony-stimulating factors.

Table 2. Characterization of *Leishmania* T-cell lines

T-Cell lines	Antigen specificity		$CD4^+$ Type	Protection
	Fraction 1	Fraction 9		
1.1	+	−	T_{H^2}	No
9.2	+	−	T_{H^2}	No
1.2	+	−	T_{H^2}	?
9A	−	+	T_{H^1}	Yes
9B	−	+	T_{H^1}	Yes
9.1	−	+	T_{H^1}	Yes
9.3	−	+	T_{H^1}	?
9.3γ	−	+	T_{H^1}	?
9.1-2	−	+	T_{H^1}	Yes

T-cell lines were obtained as described in SCOTT et al. (1988a). Antigen specificity was assayed by lymphocyte proliferation. T_{H1} and T_{H2} characterization was based on production of IL-2, IL-4, IL-5, and IFN-γ, which were measured as described in SCOTT et al. (1988a). Protection was determined by adoptive transfer experiments as described in SCOTT et al. (1988a).

The first protective T-cell line in cutaneous leishmaniasis was derived from animals protectively immunized with the semipurified antigen, fraction 9 (discussed above; SCOTT et al. 1988a). Cells from this line, line 9, transferred protection equivalent to or better than that obtained by active immunization. In contrast, a cell line recognizing the nonprotective antigens contained in fraction 1, designated line 1, exacerbated subsequent lesion development when transferred into BALB/c mice. Most importantly, when the lymphokine profile of these lines were determined, it was found that line 9 contained predominantly T_{H1} cells while line 1 contained T_{H2} cells (SCOTT et al. 1988a). These results prove that T_{H1} cells can in fact mediate protection, and that T_{H2} cells mediate susceptibility, as was suggested by the correlation between the presence of these cell types and the outcome of infection (HEINZEL et al. 1989; Table 1). In addition, however, they also suggest that different antigens may preferentially stimulate different T-cell subsets. In this regard, it was found that the correlation between antigen specificity and T_{H1}/T_{H2} development was not confined to these two cell lines and could be reliably reproduced (Table 2). The basis of this antigen bias toward particular T_H subsets is unknown. However, the possibility that different parasite antigens may lead to protective or nonprotective immune responses has been postulated in other leishmanial systems. For example, the leishmanial LPG is protective, while the glycoconjugate derived from this molecule exacerbates lesion development. It has been postulated that these results are due to the presence of protective and suppressogenic epitopes on the LPG (MITCHELL 1984). In human studies, AKUFFO et al. (1988) have suggested that parasite isolates from diffuse cutaneous leishmaniasis patients contain antigens that suppress protective immune responses, although the nature of the T cells stimulated by these antigens has not been investigated.

Protective T-cell lines have also been described in experimental visceral leishmaniasis. Thus, a T-cell line that protects against *L. donovani* infection in BALB/c mice was isolated from chronically infected animals following drug treatment (HOLADAY et al. 1988). These cells were $L3T4^+$ and produced IFN-γ, suggesting that they belong to the $T_H{}^1$-cell subset. In contrast, a cell line from animals subcutaneously immunized failed to provide protection and did not produce IFN-γ.

3.3 Protective T-Cell Clones and Identification of T-Cell Antigens

In the past it has been difficult to identify antigens recognized by T cells from protected animals. However, it is now possible to characterize the antigens recognized by T cells using the T-cell immunoblotting technique (YOUNG and LAMB 1986). With cutaneous patients, it has been demonstrated that the T-cell response to *Leishmania* is very heterogeneous (MELBY and SACKS 1987). Similarly, in both visceral and cutaneous murine models, the T-cell response is diverse (KAYE et al. 1987; P. SCOTT, unpublished data).

One of the most important uses of T-cell immunoblotting is the identification of antigens recognized by protective T-cell lines and clones. The protective T-cell line made against fraction 9 recognized antigens in the molecular weight regions of 10–12 kDa, 23–35 kDa, and 50–68 kDa. More important, however, is the development of T-cell clones that are protective. To develop such cells, line 9 was cloned by limiting dilution, and a clone, designated 9.1-2, was obtained (SCOTT et al. 1988b). This clone was capable of transferring protection equivalent to that obtained with the uncloned cell line (SCOTT et al. 1989). When the antigen specificity of this clone was assayed by T-cell immunoblotting, it was found to recognize a protein of approximate molecular weight, 10 kDa. This molecule is obviously a good candidate as a vaccine immunogen.

Another T-cell clone with presumably a different antigen specificity than clone 9.1-2 also transfers protection in the *L. major*–BALB/c model. These cells were isolated from spleens of intravenously infected mice 2 weeks after infection (MULLER et al. 1989). In vitro, they were stimulated with live *L. major* promastigotes but failed to respond to killed promastigotes or any dead antigen preparation tested. In contrast, T-cell lines made with dead parasite antigens were all found to exacerbate lesion development. MULLER et al. (1989) suggest that these results indicate that protective and nonprotective T cells may respond to distinct antigens, as is suggested by the differential responses to SLA fractions 1 and 9 (Table 2).

4 Conclusions

Experimental murine infection provides an excellent model for defining immunologic effector mechanisms in leishmaniasis. These studies have clearly shown that differential stimulation of $CD4^+$ T-cell subsets can dramatically influence the outcome of infection. In addition, they provide a model with which to rationally design and test potential leishmanial immunogens. The availability of such models will be crucial if, as is suggested by MULLER et al. (1989), not all IFN-γ producing T

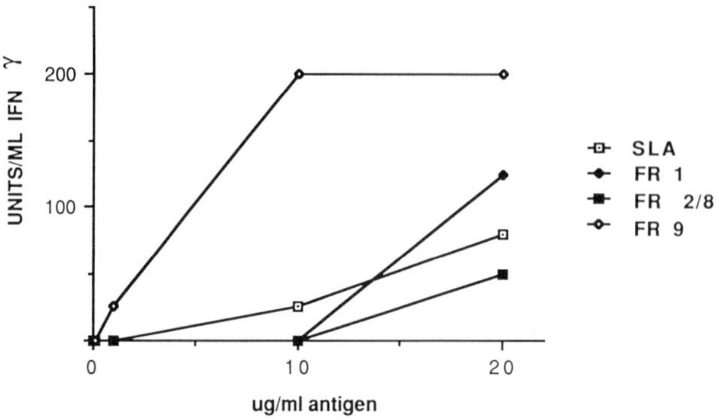

Fig. 4. IFN-γ response of a *L. major* patient to SLA fractions. Peripheral blood lymphocytes were isolated from a *L. major* patient and cultured with various concentrations of SLA or fractions derived from SLA (Scott et al. 1987b). Supernatants were harvested from the cultures on day 3, and IFN-γ was assayed using a cytopathic effect inhibition assay with vesicular stomatitis virus in WISH cells

cells are capable of inducing protection. Some of the questions yet to be answered are how and why T_{H1} and T_{H2} cells are preferentially stimulated in resistant and susceptible mice; do certain leishmanial antigens preferentially stimulate one type of $CD4^+$ T-cell, and why; whether one can reproducibly immunize with defined antigens subcutaneously; and what is the role of $CD8^+$ cells in resistance?

Possibly the most important question is how these experimental results relate to human leishmaniasis. For the most part, this is an unanswered question. The division of $CD4^+$ T cells may not be as clear-cut in man. While evidence exists that human $CD4^+$ cells can be roughly divided into the same subsets as in the mouse, T-cell clones that bridge these two subsets have been described (Umetsu et al. 1988; Rotteveel et al. 1988). However, since the factors involved in regulation and development of these cell subsets are still relatively undefined, this confusion may relate mostly to our lack of knowledge. Nevertheless, the most meaningful result may be the demonstration that certain lymphokines modulate the outcome of infection, since it is through lymphokine production that T cells function. Finally, recognition by human patients of protective antigens identified in experimental murine models will need to be tested, since it can not be assumed that protective antigens defined in mice will necessarily be recognized in man. One encouraging result in this regard is the demonstration that the protective antigens contained in fraction 9 were preferentially recognized by T cells from a patient infected with *L. major* (Fig. 4).

References

Akuffo HO, Fehniger TE, Britton S (1988) Differential recognition of *Leishmania aethiopica* antigens by lymphocytes from patients with local and diffuse cutaneous leishmaniasis. Evidence for antigen induced immune suppression. J Immunol 141: 2461–2466

Alexander J (1982) A radioattenuated *Leishmania major* vaccine markedly increases the resistance of CBA mice to subsequent infection with *Leishmania mexicana mexicana*. Trans R Soc Trop Med Hyg 76: 646–649

Anderson S, David JR, McMahon-Pratt D (1983) In vivo protection against *Leishmania mexicana* mediated by monoclonal antibodies. J Immunol 131: 1616–1618

Badaro R, Jones TC, Carvalho EM, Sampaio D, Reed SG, Barral A, Teixeira R, Johnson WD Jr (1986) New perspectives on a subclinical form of visceral leishmaniasis. J Infect Dis 154: 1003–1011

Behin RJ, Mauel J, Sordat B (1979) *Leishmania tropica*: pathogenicity and in vitro macrophage function in strains of inbred mice. Exp Parasitol 48: 81–91

Belosevic M, Finbloom DS, van der Meide P, Slayter MZ, Nacy CA (1989) Administration of monoclonal anti-IFN-γ antibodies in vivo abrogates natural resistance of C3H/HeN mice to infection with *Leishmania major*. J Immunol 143: 266–274

Blackwell JM, Ulczak OM (1984) Immunoregulation of genetically controlled acquired responses to *Leishmania donovani* infection in mice: demonstration and characterization of suppressor T cells in non-cure mice. Infect Immun 44: 97–102

Blackwell J, Freeman J, Bradley D (1980) Influence of H-2 complex on acquired resistance to *Leishmania donovani* infection in mice. Nature 283: 72–74

Bradley DJ, Kirkley J (1977) Regulation of *Leishmania* populations within the host. I. The variable course of *Leishmania donovani* infection in mice. Clin Exp Immunol 30: 119–129

Button LL, McMaster WR (1988) Molecular cloning of the major surface antigen of *Leishmania*. J Exp Med 167: 724–729

Champsi J, McMahon-Pratt D (1988) Membrane glycoprotein M-2 protects against *Leishmania amazonensis* infection. Infect Immun 52: 3272–3279

Chang CS, Chang KP (1986) Monoclonal antibody affinity purification of a *Leishmania* membrane glycoprotein and its inhibition of *Leishmania*-macrophage binding. Proc Natl Acad Sci USA 83: 100–104

Coutinho SG, Louis JA, Mauel J, Engers HD (1984) Induction of specific T Lymphocytes of intracellular destruction of *Leishmania major* in infected murine macrophages. Parasite Immunol 6: 157–169

DeTolla LJ, Scott PA, Farrell JP (1981) Single gene control of resistance to cutaneous leishmaniasis in mice. Immunogenetics 14: 29–39

Etges RJ, Bouvier J, Hoffman R, Bordier C (1985) Evidence that the major surface proteins of three *Leishmania* species are structurally related. Mol Biochem Parasitol 14; 141–149

Farrell JP, Muller I, Louis JA (1989) A role for Lyt 2^+ T cells in resistance to cutaneous leishmaniasis in immunized mice. J Immunol 142: 2052–2056

Feng ZY, Louis JA , Kindler V, Pedrazzini T, Eliason J, Behin R, Vassalli P (1988) Aggravation of experimental cutaneous leishmaniasis in mice by administration of interleukin-3. Eur J Immunol 18: 1245–1251

Frommel D, Ogunkolade BW, Vouldoukis I, Monjour L (1988) Vaccine induced immunity against cutaneous leishmaniasis in BALB/c mice. Infect Immun 56: 843–848

Greenblatt CL (1980) The present and future of vaccination for cutaneous leishmaniasis. In: Hertman AI, Kohn A et al. (eds) In: New developments with human and veterinary vaccines. New York, pp 259–285 (Progress in clinical and biological research, vol 47)

Greene MI, Benacerraf B (1980) Studies on hapten specific T cell immunity and suppression. Immunol Rev 50: 163–186

Greil J, Bodendorffer B, Rollinghoff M, Solbach W (1988) Application of recombinant granulocyte-macrophage colony-stimulating factor has a detrimental effect in experimental murine leishmaniasis. Eur J Immunol 18: 1527–1533

Handman E, Goding JW (1985) The *Leishmania* receptor for macrophages is a lipid containing glycoconjugate. EMBO J 4: 329–336

Handman E, Hocking E (1982) Stage-specific, strain-specific and cross reactive antigens of *Leishmania* species identified by monoclonal antibodies. Infect Immun 37: 28–33

Handman E, Mitchell GF (1985) Immunization with *Leishmania* receptor macrophages protects mice against cutaneous leishmaniasis. Proc Natl Acad Sci USA 82: 5910–5914

Handman E, Ceredig R, Mitchell GF (1979) Murine cutaneous leishmaniasis: disease patterns in intact and nude mice of various genotypes and examination of some differences between normal and infected macrophages. Aust J Exp Biol Med Sci 57: 9–29

Heinzel FP, Sadick MD, Locksley RM (1988) *Leishmania major*: analysis of lymphocyte and macrophage cellular phenotypes during infection of susceptible and resistant mice. Exp Parasitol 65: 258–269

Heinzel FP, Sadick MD, Holaday BJ, Coffman RL, Locksley RM (1989) Reciprocal expression of interferon gamma or interleukin 4 during the resolution or progression of murine leishmaniasis. J Exp Med 169: 59–72

Holaday B, Sadick MD, Pearson RD (1988) Isolation of protective T cells from BALB/cJ mice chronically infected with *Leishmania donovani*. J Immunol 141: 2132–2137

Hoover DL, Nacy CA (1984) Macrophage activation to kill *Leishmania tropica*: defective intracellular killing of amastigotes by macrophages elicited with sterile inflammatory agents. J Immunol 132: 1487–1493
Howard JG (1986) Immunologic regulation and control of experimental leishmaniasis. Int Rev Exp Pathol 28: 79–116
Howard JG, Hale C, Liew FY (1980) Immunologic regulation of experimental cutaneous leishmaniasis. I. Immunogenetic aspects of susceptibility to *Leishmania tropica* in mice. Parasite Immunol 2: 303–314
Howard JG, Hale C, Liew FY (1981) Immunologic regulation of experimental cutaneous leishmaniasis. IV. Prophylactic effect of sublethal irradiation as a result of abrogation of suppressor T cell generation in mice genetically susceptible to *Leishmania tropica*. J Exp Med 153: 557–568
Howard JG, Nicklin S, Hale C, Liew FY (1982) Prophylactic immunization against experimental leishmaniasis. I. Protection induced in mice genetically vulnerable to fatal *Leishmania tropica* infection. J. Immunol 129: 2206–2212
Howard JG, Liew FY, Hale C, Nicklin S (1984) Prophylactic immunization against experimental leishmaniasis. II. Further characterization of the protective immunity against fatal *Leishmania tropica* infection induced by irradiated promastigotes. J Immunol 132: 450–461
Kaufmann SHE (1988) $CD8^+$ T lymphocytes in intracellular microbial infections. Immunol Today 9: 168–174
Kaye PM, Roberts MB, Blackwell JM (1987) Analysing the immune response to *Leishmania donovani* infection. Ann Inst Pasteur Immunol 138: 737–795
Kirkpatrick CE, Farrell JP, Warner JF, Denner G (1985) Participation of natural killer cells in the recovery of mice from visceral leishmaniasis. Cell Immunol 92: 163–171
Lelchuk R, Graveley R, Liew FY (1988) Susceptibility to murine cutaneous leishmaniasis correlates with the capacity to generate interleukin 3 in response to *Leishmania* antigen in vitro. Cell Immunol 111: 66–76
Liew FY (1987) Analysis of host-protective and disease promoting T cells. Ann Inst Pasteur Immunol 138: 749–755
Liew FY, Hale C, Howard JG (1982) Immunologic regulation of experimental cutaneous leishmaniasis. V. Characterization of effector and specific suppressor T cells. J Immunol 128: 1917–1922
Liew FY, Singleton A, Cillari E, Howard JG (1985a) Prophylactic immunization against experimental leishmaniasis. V. Mechanism of the anti-protective blocking effect induced by subcutaneous immunization against *Leishmania major* infection. J Immunol 135: 2102–2107
Liew FY, Hale C, Howard JG (1985b) Prophylactic immunization against experimental leishmaniasis. IV. Subcutaneous immunization prevents the induction of protective immunity against fatal *Leishmania major* infection. J Immunol 135: 2095–2101
Louis JA, Pedrazzini T, Titus RG, Muller I, Farrell JP, Kindler V, Vassalli P, Marchal G, Milon G (1987) Subsets of specific T cells and experimental cutaneous leishmaniasis. Ann Inst Pasteur Immunol 138: 755–758
McElrath JM, Kaplan G, Nusrat A, Cohn Z (1987) Cutaneous leishmaniasis. The defect in T cell influx in BALB/c mice. J Exp Med 165: 546–559
Melby PC, Sacks DL (1987) Analysis of the heterogeneity of T cell responses in human leishmaniasis. Ann Inst Pasteur Immunol 138: 768–771
Milon G, Titus RG, Cerrottini J-C, Marchal G, Louis JA (1986) Higher frequency of *Lishmania major* specific $L3T4^+$ cells in susceptible BALB/c as compared to resistant CBA mice. J Immunol 136: 1467–1471
Mirkovich A, Galelli A, Allison AC, Modabber FZ (1986) Increased myelopoiesis during *L. major* infection in mice: generation of safe targets, a possible way to evade the effector immune mechanism. Clin Exp Immunol 64: 1–7
Mitchell GF (1984) Host protection and its suppression in a parasitic disease: murine cutaneous leishmaniasis. Immunol Today 5: 224–226
Mitchell GF, Handman E (1986) The glycoconjugate derived from a *Leishmania major* receptor for macrophages is a suppressogenic disease promoting antigen in murine cutaneous leishmaniasis. Parasite Immunol 8: 255–263
Mitchell GF, Curtis JM, Handman E, McKenzie IFC (1980) Cutaneous leishmaniasis in mice: disease patterns in reconstitutge nude mice of several genotypes infected with *Leishmania tropica*. Aust J Exp Med Biol Sci 58: 521–532
Mitchell GF, Curtis JM, Scollay RG, Handman E (1981a) Resistance and abrogation of resistance to cutaneous leishmaniasis in reconstituted BALB/c nude mice. Aust J Exp Med Biol Sci 59: 539–554
Mitchell GF, Curtis JM, Handman E (1981b) Resistance to cutaneous leishmaniasis in genetically susceptible BALB/c mice. Aust J Exp Med Biol Sci 59: 555–565
Mosmann TR, Cherwinski H, Bond MW, Giedlin MA, Coffman RL (1986) Two types of murine helper T

cell clone. J. Definition according to profiles of lymphokine activities and secreted proteins. J Immunol 136: 2348–2357
Muller I, Louis JA (1989) Immunity to experimental infection with *Leishmania majors* generation of protective L3T4 + T cell clones recognizing antigen(s) associated with live parasites. Eur J Immunol 19: 865–872
Muller I, Pedrazzini T, Farrell JP, Louis J (1989) T cell responses and immunity to experimental infection with *Leishmania major*. Annu Rev Immunol 7: 561–578
Murray HW, Masur H, Keithly JS (1982) Cell mediated immune response in experimental visceral leishmaniasis. I. Correlation between resistance to *Leishmania donovani* and lymphokine generating capacity. J Immunol 129: 344–350
Murray HW, Rubin BY, Rothermal CD (1983) Killing of intracellular *Leishmania donovani* by lymphokine-stimulated human mononuclear phagocytes: evidence that interferon gamma is the activating lymphokine. J Clin Invest 72: 1506–1510
Murray HW, Stern JJ, Welte K, Rubin BY, Carriero SM, Nathan CF (1987) Experimental visceral leishmaniasis: production of interleukin 2 and interferon gamma, tissue immune reaction, and response to treatment with interleukin-2 and interferon gamma. J Immunol 138: 2290–2297
Nacy CA, Meltzer MS, Lenoard EJ, Wyler DJ (1981) Intracellular replication and lymphokine induced destruction of *Leishmania tropica* in C3H/HeN mouse macrophages. J Immunol 127: 2381–2386
Nacy CA, Fortier AH, Pappas MG, Henry R (1983) Susceptibility of inbred mice to *Leishmania* infection: correlation of susceptibility with in vitro defective macrophage microbicidal activities. Cell Immunol 77: 298–307
Panosian CB, Sypek JP, Wyler DJ (1984) Cell contact mediated macrophage activation for antileishmanial defense. I. Lymphocyte effector mechanism that is contact dependent and noncytotoxic. J Immunol 127: 3358–3365
Preston PM, Carter RL, Leuchars E, Davies AJS, Dumonde DC (1972) Experimental cutaneous leishmaniasis. III. Effect of thymectomy on the course of infection of CBA mice with *Leishmania tropica*. Clin Exp Immunol 10: 337–357
Rezai HR, Farrell JP, Soulsby EL (1980) Immunologic responses of *Leishmania donovani* infection in mice and significance of T cell resistance to experimental leishmaniasis. Clin Exp Immunol 40: 508–514
Rodrigues MM, Mendonca-Previato L, Charlab R, Barcinski M (1987) The cellular immune response to a purified antigen from *Leishmania mexicana subsp. amizonensis* enhances the size of the leishmanial lesion on susceptible mice. Infect Immun 55: 3142–3148
Rotteveel FTM, Kokkelink I, van Lier RAW, Kuenen B, Meager A, Miedema F, Lucas CJ (1988) Clonal analysis of functionally distinct human $CD4^+$ T cell subsets. J Exp Med 168: 1659–1673
Russell DG, Alexander J (1988) Effective immunization against cutaneous leishmaniasis with defined membrane antigens reconstituted into liposomes. J Immunol 140: 1274–1279
Russell DG, Wilhelm H (1986) The involvement of the major surface glycoprotein (gp63) of *Leishmania* promastigotes in attachment to macrophages. J Immunol 136: 2613–2620
Sadick MD, Locksley RM, Tubbs C, Raff HV (1986) Murine cutaneous leishmaniasis: resistance correlates with the capacity to generate interferon-gamma in response to *Leishmania* antigens in vitro. J Immunol 136: 655–661
Scott PA, Farrell JP (1981) Experimental cutaneous leishmaniasis. I. Non-specific immunodepression in BALB/c mice infected with *Leishmania tropica*. J Immunol 127: 2395–2400
Scott P, Sher A (1986) A spectrum in the susceptibility of leishmanial strains to intracellular killing by murine macrophages. J Immunol 136: 1461–1466
Scott P, Natovitz P, Sher A (1986) B lymphocytes are required for the generation of T cells that mediate healing of cutaneous leishmaniasis. J Immunol 137: 1017–1021
Scott P, Pearce E, Natovitz P, Sher A (1987a) Vaccination against cutaneous leishmaniasis in a murine model. I. Induction of protective immunity with a soluble extract of promastigotes. J Immunol 139: 221–227
Scott P, Pearce E, Natovitz P, Sher A (1987b) Vaccination against cutaneous leishmaniasis in a murine model. II. Immunologic properties of protective and nonprotective subfractions of a soluble promastigote extract. J Immunol 139: 3118–3125
Scott P, Natovitz P, Coffman RL, Pearce E, Sher A (1988a) Immunoregulation of cutaneous leishmaniasis. T cell lines that transfer protective immunity or exacerbation belong to different T helper subsets and respond to distinct parasite antigens. J Exp Med 168: 1675–1684
Scott P, Pearce E, Natovitz P, Sher A (1988b) An approach for identifying protective leishmanial antigens by T cell cloning and immunoblotting. In: Ginsberg H, Brown F, Lernee RA, Chanock RM (eds) Vaccines 88. Cold Spring Harbor Laboratory, Cold Spring Harbor NY, pp 57–60

Scott P, Caspar P, Sher A (1989) Protection against *Leishmania major* in BALB/c mice by adoptive transfer of a T cell clone recognizing a low molecular weight antigen released by promastigotes. J Immunol, in press

Solbach W, Lohoff M, Streck H, Rohner P, Rollinghoff M (1987) Kinetics of cell mediated immunity developing during the course of *Leishmania major* infection in healer and non-healer mice: progressive impairment of response to and generation of interleukin 2. Immunology 62: 485–492

Stern JJ, Oca MJ, Rubin BY, Anderson SL, Murray HW (1988) Role of $L3T4^+$ and $Lyt\text{-}2^+$ T cells in experimental visceral leishmaniasis. J Immunol 140: 3971–3977

Titus RG, Lima GC, Engers HD, Louis JA (1984) Exacerbation of murine cutaneous leishmaniasis by adoptive transfer of parasite specific helper T cell populations capable of mediating *Leishmania major* specific delayed type hypersensitivity. J Immunol 133: 1594–1600

Titus RG, Ceredig R, Cerrottini JC, Louis JA (1985) Therapeutic effect of anti-L3T4 monoclonal antibody GK 1.5 on cutaneous leishmaniasis in genetically susceptible BALB/c mice. J Immunol 135: 2108–2114

Titus RG, Milon G, Marchal G, Vassalli P, Cerottini JC, Louis JA (1987) Involvement of specific $Lyt\text{-}2^+$ T cells in the immunologic control of experimentally induced murine cutaneous leishmaniasis. Eur J Immunol 17: 1429–1433

Umetsu DT, Jabara HH, DeKruyff RH, Abbas AK, Abrams JS, Geha RS (1988) Functional heterogeneity among human inducer T cell clones. J Immunol 140: 4211–4216

Wyler DJ, Beller DI, Sypek JP (1987) Macrophage activation for anti-leishmanial defense by an apparently novel mechanism. J Immunol 138: 1246–1249

Young DB, Lamb JR (1986) T lymphocytes respond to solid phase antigen: a novel approach to the molecular analysis of cellular immunity. Immunology 59: 167–171

Regulation of Cell-Mediated Immunity in Leishmaniasis

F. Y. LIEW

1 Leishmaniasis

Leishmaniasis is caused by species of the intracellular protozoan parasite belonging to the genus *Leishmania*. There are three main categories of leishmaniasis: cutaneous leishmaniasis (oriental sore), mucocutaneous leishmaniasis (espundia) and visceral leishmaniasis (kala azar). An incidence rate of 400 000 new cases per year has been reported, and the world wide prevalence of leishmaniasis is estimated to be 12 million cases (MODABBER 1987). Visceral leishmaniasis is fatal if not treated. The last epidemic of leishmaniasis that occurred in India in 1977–1978 caused an estimated 20 000 deaths. Most forms of leishmaniasis are zoonotic, and humans are infected only secondarily. Animal reservoirs of species pathogenic to man include the sloth, dog and rodent. The parasites are transmitted by female sandflies, and the flagellated promastigotes develop in the gut of the sandfly and in cell-free cultures. Transformation into the amastigote stage occurs within the mammalian macrophage. Primary drug treatment is based on antimony compounds, notably the pentavalent antimonials sodium stibogluconate and *N*-methylglucamine antimonate. These must be given in daily intramuscular doses for several weeks; they entail unpleasant side effects and are not very effective against cutaneous leishmaniasis. The only immunisation strategy against leishmaniasis used so far with any success in man has been restricted to the cutaneous diseases. It is based on convalescent immunity following controlled induction of a lesion with viable *L. major* (GREENBLATT 1980). The feasibility of vaccination with killed vaccines is currently being evaluated.

The use of inbred mouse strains has greatly advanced our understanding of the immunological control of leishmaniasis. Mice are susceptible to most species of leishmania that are pathogenic to man, and a spectrum of disease pattern can be obtained according to the genetic background of the host. In the case of visceral leishmaniasis (caused by *L. donovani*) the innate susceptibility is determined by the *Lsh* gene (BRADLEY 1977; BLACKWELL 1983) in the mouse chromosome 1, whilst the acquired immunity is controlled by at least three additional genes: H-2 linked *Rld*-1,

Department of Experimental Immunobiology, Wellcome Research Laboratories, Beckenham, Kent BR3 3BS, UK

Current Topics in Microbiology and Immunology, Vol. 155

H-11 linked and Ir-2 linked genes. In cutaneous leishmaniasis, the distinction between innate and acquired resistance is less clear, but the susceptibility of inbred mice to *L. major* infection is controlled by *Scl*-1, *Scl*-2 (BLACKWELL et al. 1985a) and H-11 linked genes (BLACKWELL et al. 1985b). Involvement of the H-2 linked gene is relatively minor. The phenotypic expression of these genes is at present unknown, but the *Lsh* gene appears to determine the ability of Kupffer's cells to eliminate intracellular *L. donovani* (CROCKER et al. 1987) whilst the susceptibility/resistance to *L. major* is adoptively transferable by the bone marrow cells in H-2 compatible radiation chimaeras (HOWARD et al. 1980).

2 Cell-Mediated Immunity in Leishmaniasis

Cell-mediated immunity (CMI) rather than humoral antibody plays a causal role in the acquired immunity to leishmaniasis. Anti-leishmanial antibodies have been shown in vitro to lyse promastigotes in the presence of complement (PEARSON and STEIGBIGEL 1980) and to promote phagocytosis (HERMAN 1980). However, there is little evidence for a corresponding in vivo role for antibody in determining the outcome of leishmanial infection. Treatment of mice from birth with anti-IgM antibody can profoundly affect the outcome of *L. major* infections (SACKS et al. 1984; SCOTT et al. 1986). This effect is likely to be due to the depletion of the antigen-presenting function of B cells rather than the abrogation of antibody production, since reconstitution with specific antibody could not restore the effects of the anti-IgM treatment (F.Y. LIEW et al., unpublished).

In contrast to humoral immunity, the case for a causal role of CMI in acquired resistance to leishmaniasis is based on a range of impressive clinical and experimental evidence (Reviewed in LIEW 1986). Resistant CBA mice rendered relatively T-cell deficient by thymectomy followed by irradiation and reconstitution with syngeneic bone marrow cells are less able to control *L. major* infection (PRESTON et al. 1972). Athymic mutants of the highly resistant CBA and C57BL mice are totally unable to control *L. major* infection which progresses and visceralises. Normal resistance, however, can be fully restored by reconstitution with normal syngeneic T cells (MITCHELL et al. 1981). Acquired immunity against *L. major* (PRESTON and DUMONDE 1976) and *L. donovani* (REZAI et al. 1980) as a result of recovery from infection or prophylactic immunisation can also be transferred by T cells but not B-cells (LIEW et al. 1984). Treatment of resistant C3H mice from birth with anti-IgM antibody rendered them defective in antibody response and also susceptible to *L. major* infection. However, lesion progression in these treated mice can be arrested and the disease outcome reversed by adoptive transfer of T cells alone from normal C3H donors without any restoration of humoral antibody formation (SCOTT et al. 1986). These results therefore provide a forceful argument for a pivotal role of CMI in acquired resistance to leishmaniasis.

There now appears to be a broad consensus that T cells conferring protective immunity primarily belong to the $CD4^+$ subset. This is supported by experimental evidence from several laboratories using adoptive transfer and replacement studies with the murine *L. major* (MITCHELL et al. 1981; LIEW et al. 1982) or *L. mexicana* (GORCZYNSKI 1985) models. Lymphokines such as macrophage-activating factor (MAF) and interferon-gamma (IFN-γ) produced by specifically sensitised T cells are deemed to be essential for the activation of infected macrophages to eliminate intracellular amastigotes (MAUEL and BEHIN 1982).

Recent evidence suggests that $CD8^+$ T cells may also be protective against *L. major* infection (TITUS et al. 1987). Resistant CBA mice became less able to heal from *L. major* infection after repeated CD8 monoclonal antibody treatment in vivo. However, the effect of CD8 monoclonal antibody treatment was far less impressive than that of CD4. The extreme susceptibility of athymic nude BALB/c mice to *L. donovani* infection could only be reversed by a combination of $CD4^+$ and $CD8^+$ T cells. Each cell population alone failed to reconstitute the athymic mice to the resistant status of their euthymic litter mates (STERN et al. 1988). However, thus far, $CD8^+$-specific cytotoxic T cells have not been convincingly demonstrated in leishmaniasis. The efficacy of cytotoxic T cells against infectious agents is based primarily on the destruction of host cell containing replicating pathogens which when released prematurely could not survive in the host's environment or fail to reinfect other host cells. This generally works well against obligatory intracellular infectious agents such as viruses. However, few protozoa or helminths have such limitations. Therefore, it is not clear at this stage whether the protective role of $CD8^+$ T cells in protozoa infections rests on their cytolytic capacity or the lymphokines secreted by them.

3 Impairment of Protective Immunity

Specific and generalised immune suppression has been reported in a number of acute and chronic infections. From an evolutionary view point, a self-regulatory suppressive mechanism is essential during *Trypanosoma cruzi* infection to maintain a fine balance between resistance to infection and autoimmunity. In leishmaniasis, both specific and non-specific immune suppression were evident in mice and individuals susceptible to leishmaniasis. Clinically, patients with visceral leishmaniasis do not develop leishmanial-specific skin reaction or proliferative T-cell response (REZAI et al. 1978; HO et al. 1983). These reactions are restored following successful chemotherapy (CARVALHO et al. 1981; HALDAR et al. 1983). In experimental models, the reduced spleen cell activation by pythohaemagglutinin during *L. donovani* infection in BALB/c mice compared with that of normal controls is associated with impaired interleukin 2 (IL-2) production (REINER and FINKE 1983). The depressed mitogen-induced cellular proliferation and IL-2 production in mice susceptible to *L. major* infection is attributable to the presence of a population of macrophage-like adherent suppressor cells (SCOTT and FARRELL 1981; CILLARI et al. 1986). A similar non-specific suppression of IL-2 production in clinical visceral leishmaniasis has also been demonstrated (PETERSON et al. 1984; CILLARI et al. 1988).

The suppression of IL-2 production appears to be mediated by macrophages and is pronounced only at the terminal stages of infection (SCOTT and FARRELL 1981; CILLARI et al. 1986). In contrast, the antigen-specific suppression of delayed-type hypersensitivity (DTH) occurs earlier and is mediated by $CD4^+$ T cells. There has been much controversy over the identity of these $CD4^+$ suppressor cells because they do not have the conventional $CD8^+$ suppressor T-cell phenotype, and their supressive activity is defined mainly in operational terms. Recent studies clearly demonstrate that the suppressor T (Ts) cells described earlier are not the conventional Ts cells, although operationally they interfere with the host protective immunity. Studies leading to this conclusion are described below.

The majority of inbred mouse strains are resistant to *L. major* infections. BALB/c mice, however, are exceptionally susceptible to this infection in that they develop uniformly fatal disseminating disease even with a minimal infecting dose. The failure of BALB/c mice to contain *L. major* infection is not due to any intrinsic inability of these mice to develop effective $CD4^+$ T cells against the parasites. In fact, BALB/c mice can be rendered resistant to *L. major* infection by prior sublethal whole body γ-irradiation (HOWARD et al. 1981), treatment from birth with anti-μ antibody (SACKS et al. 1984), injection with CD4 monoclonal antibody (TITUS et al. 1985) or cyclosporin A (BEHFOROUZ et al. 1986; SOLBACH et al. 1986). The recovered mice develop a classical tuberculin-type of DTH (footpad swelling begins at 10 h and is sustained to 48 h after injection), and their splenic and lymph node T cells can adoptively transfer resistance in otherwise highly susceptible BALB/c recipients (LIEW and DHALIWAL 1987). The protective T cells, like those found in the recovered resistant mice, are $CD4^+$ and produce MAF or IFN-γ when cultured with leishmanial antigens in vitro (LIEW and DHALIWAL 1987).

The prophylactic effect of sublethal irradiation or anti-μ treatment can be reversed by the injection into these treated BALB/c mice with T cells from normal syngeneic T cells or, even more readily, T cells from mice with progressive *L. major* infection (HOWARD et al. 1981). At a population level, the disease-promoting T cells (operationally called Ts cells) from mice with progressive disease are functionally opposite to the protective T cells obtained from recovered mice (here referred to as Tr cells; Table I). These Ts cells also express the $CD4^+$ phenotype. They are extremely potent; as few as 10^6 cells can reverse the disease-resisting capability of γ-irradiated BALB/c mice. The Ts cells do not mediate the classical tuberculin DTH (LIEW and DHALIWAL 1987). Instead, they can suppress the expression of classical DTH of Tr cells (LIEW 1983). What then are the characteristics and mechanism of interaction between the Tr cells and the Ts cells, both of which are $CD4^+$?

4 Heterogeneity of $CD4^+$ T Cells

Since both the host-protection and the disease-promotion are mediated by $CD4^+$ T cells, it has been argued that the two phenomena are the function of the same population of T cells. The difference merely reflects a differential quantitative requirement of the helper T cells (TITUS et al. 1984; LOUIS et al. 1986). In other words, too many protective T cells are detrimental, a suggestion reminiscent of the 'too much help leads to suppression' concept. However, recent reports have provided compelling evidence that the disease-promoting $CD4^+$ T cells are functionally distinct from the host-protective $CD4^+$ T cells. Firstly, freshly isolated T cells from mice with progressive disease either exacerbate disease ($>10^7$ cells per recipient) or have no effect ($<10^7$ cells per recipient). No protection was offerred at any dose. Conversely, freshly isolated T cells from mice recovered from infection are either protective ($>10^7$ cells per recipient) or ineffective ($<10^7$ cells per recipient). No disease exacerbation was observed at any dose (LIEW et al. 1987). Secondly, T cells derived from resistant strains of mice or protected BALB/c mice secrete IFN-γ in response to leishmanial antigens, whereas T cells that promote disease are devoid of such activity (SADICK et al. 1986; LIEW and DHALIWAL 1987). Thirdly, the disease-promoting T cells produce IL-3 (LELCHUK et al. 1988), IL-4 and IL-5 (SCOTT et al. 1988a). When the abundance of lymphokine-specific mRNA in the lymph node cells of *L. major*-infected mice with healer and non-healer phenotypes were examined, IFN-γ mRNA correlated with protection whilst IL-4 mRNA correlated with progressive disease (HEINZEL et al. 1989). Finally, the most direct evidence was provided by T-cell clones. A $CD4^+$ T-cell clone was derived from BALB/c mice with potential to develop exacerbated *L. major* infection (TITUS et al. 1984). The cell line significantly enhanced disease development in recipient mice infected with *L. major*. Recently, T cells from BALB/c mice protectively immunised with chemically mutagenised avirulent clones of *L. major* (TITUS et al. 1988) or purified *L. major* antigen (SCOTT et al. 1988b) were cloned. These $CD4^+$ T cell clones can adoptively transfer protection.

$CD4^+$ T cells are involved in a variety of activities, including antigen-specific or polyclonal B-cell activation, DTH, killing of appropriate target cells, suppression of DTH and antibody responses, and induction of $CD8^+$ killer or suppressor T cells. Early studies showed that T cells mediating help for antibody synthesis in the carrier-hapten system are distinct from those involved in the DTH to the carrier protein (LIEW and PARISH 1974; SILVER and BENACERRAF 1974). Furthermore, there appears a direct correlation between DTH reactivity and high-, and low-zone tolerance to antibody synthesis (PARISH and LIEW 1972). These early findings strongly imply a functional heterogeneity of $CD4^+$ T cells. Later studies also suggest the presence of two distinct types of $CD4^+$ cells (T_{H1} and T_{H2}) providing help to B cells (MARRACK and KAPPLER 1975; JANEWAY 1975). However, the heterogeneity of $CD4^+$ T cells was firmly established only after the discovery that $CD4^+$ T cells can be subdivided according to the expression of restricted populations of CD45 molecules (MORIMOTO et al. 1985; ARTHUR and MASON 1986; the leukocyte common antigens, T200), and that different $CD4^+$ T cell clones may secrete distinct lymphokines (MOSMANN et al. 1986).

The heterogeneity of $CD4^+$ T cells in humans and rats, and other systems in mice, has been recently reviewed (MOSMANN and COFFMAN 1987; BOTTOMLY 1988; POWRIE and MASON 1988). The comparison between the leishmanial and the other murine systems in terms of information available for leishmaniasis is summarised in Table 1. Based on lymphokine secretion, the protective T cells appear to fit into the T_{H1}/inflammatory cell category, whilst the counter-protective cells seem to be

Table 1. Comparison of the protective and counter-protective CD4$^+$ T cells in leishmaniasis with T_{H1} and T_{H2} cells

	T_{H1}/inflammatory[a]	Protective[b]	T_{H2}/helper	Counter-protective
Function measured				
Help for specific antibody	−	+	+	+
Cytotoxicity	+	−	−	−
DTH	+	+	−	−
Cytokines released				
IL-2	+	+	−	±
IL-3	+	−	+	+
IL-4	−	−	+	+
IFN-γ	+	+	−	−

[a]From Bottomly 1988
[b]From Liew 1989

equivalent to the T_{H2}/helper group. The exception is IL-3, which is secreted by both T_{H1} and T_{H2} cells and is produced only by the counter-protective T-cell. Functionally, however, there are several major discrepancies, including help for specific-antibody production, cytotoxicity and DTH reactivity. It should be pointed out that antigen-specific killer cells have not been clearly demonstrated in the leishmania system. The DTH response can be divided into the Jones-Mote hypersensitivity and the classical tuberculin response. These differences suggest that the heterogeneity of CD4$^+$ T cells may extend beyond the T_{H1} and T_{H2} classification. It should also be noted that the comparison shown in Table 1 is made between a mixed population of cells and cloned cell lines. More meaningful comparisons can only be carried out with established T-cell clones which reflect the functional characteristics of their progenitors in vivo.

Comparison of the CD4$^+$ T cell subsets between human, rats and mice has not been straightforward. Rat T cells have proved to be difficult to clone and attempts to find human T-cell clones that fit into the T_{H1}/T_{H2} classification have generally been unsuccessful.

In cutaneous leishmaniasis, therefore, there are at least two distinct subsets of CD4$^+$ T cells: Tr/T_{H1} and Ts/T_{H2}, the former is host protective and the latter disease promoting. The balance between these two populations of CD4$^+$ T cells appears to determine the outcome of the infection. Two major questions are obvious: (a) How are the two subsets of CD4$^+$ T cells preferentially induced? (b) How do they influence each other?

5 Induction of CD4$^+$ T Cell Subsets

Mice immunised intravenously with killed whole *L. major* promastigotes or their soluble antigen extract develop substantial resistance to a challenge infection (Howard et al. 1982). The protection is mediated by the equivalent of T_{H1} cells. In contrast, the same antigen preparations injected via the subcutaneous route are not only ineffective but induce a T_{H2}-equivalent cell population which can inhibit the induction of effective protection by the intravenous route of immunisation or transfer of immunity by the protective T cells (LIEW et al. 1985). These observations underline the crucial role of antigen presentation in the induction of $CD4^+$ T-cell subsets.

An interesting hypothesis has been put forward by MITCHELL and HANDMAN (1985) who argue that a lipid-containing glycoconjugate (L-GC) and the delipidated water soluble glycoconjugate (DL-GC) derived from *L. major* promastigotes by enzyme cleavage play a central role in murine cutaneous leishmaniasis. They proposed that L-GC, when anchored by lipid and orientated in relation to major histocompatibility complex (MHC) class II molecule on infected macrophage, would preferentially induce the protective $CD4^+$ T cells. On the other hand, DL-GC bound to macrophages via specific receptors and unassociated with MHC is thought to activate the disease-promoting $CD4^+$ T cells. Supporting this are the findings that L-GC are protective whereas DL-GC are disease-promoting when injected intraperitoneally into BALB/c mice. The hypothesis makes the assumption that the glycolipids are the dominant immunogens. However, it has not been convincingly demonstrated that highly purified glycolipids can induce or indeed be recognised by T cells. It is also clear that protein fractions of *L. major* are also potent protective immunogens (SCOTT et al. 1987; RUSSELL and ALEXANDER 1988). Alternatively, the two subsets of $CD4^+$ T cells may recognise distinct antigenic epitopes. Supporting this notion is the finding that tunicamycin-treated *L. mexicana* are no longer able to induce a protective response in BALB/c but retain the ability to stimulate suppression of protective immunity when given subcutaneously (GORCZYNSKI 1986). A T-cell line established against a soluble fraction of *L. major* antigen preparation can transfer protection equivalent to that obtained by active immunisation. In contrast, another T-cell line responsive to a non-protective soluble fraction not only failed to protect BALB/c mice against *L. major* infection but exacerbated the disease. The protective cells are equivalent to T_{H1} whilst the disease-promoting T cells are akin to T_{H2} (SCOTT et al. 1988a).

It may be that the question of preferential induction can be resolved only by detailed analysis of molecularly defined eiptopes and their association with class II MHC antigen on purified antigen-presenting cells. The possibility of inducing the two distinct subsets of T cells with leishmanial antigens by different routes of immunisation and the availability of complete amino acid sequence of some immunogenic proteins (BUTTON and MCMASTER 1988) together with the three-dimensional structure of MHC molecules should facilitate such a task. Recently a peptide of ten residues corresponding to the tandemly repeating unit of an intracellular glycoprotein (WALLIS and MCMASTER 1987) has been synthesised and tested for immunogenicity. This peptide failed to induce protective immunity but can exacerbate disease development in BALB/c mice immunised by subcutaneously route together with a wide range of adjuvants (F.Y. LIEW, J.A. SCHMIDT, S. MILLOTT, submitted). The knowledge gained in this area will be useful for rational design of vaccine in general and against leishmaniasis in particular.

6 Functional Relationship Between Different CD4$^+$ T Cells

The next important question is how do the different subsets of T cells in leishmaniasis influence each other in such a way that their balance determines the outcome of the disease. In a recent series of experiments (Liew et al. 1989) it was demonstrated that the antigen-specific culture supernatant of lymphoid cells from BALB/c mice with progressive disease can inhibit the MAF activity of the culture supernatant of lymphoid cells from mice recovered from *L. major* infection. Thus the ability of macrophages to kill a tumour cell line or intracellular leishmania parasites after culturing with the supernatant of Tr/T_{H1} cells was completely abolished if the culture also contained supernatant of Ts/T_{H2} cells. Furthermore, the active ingredient of MAF appears to be IFN-γ, whereas the MAF inhibiting factors are IL-3 and IL-4. The whole system can be reproduced with recombinant IFN-γ, IL-3 and IL-4, and the MAF inhibiting activity of the suppressive supernatant can be reversed by specific anti-IL-3 and anti-IL-4 antibodies. It thus appears that the two subsets of CD4$^+$ T cells modulate the outcome of the disease by influencing the ability of macrophage to kill the intracellular parasite. This may be a means by which the different CD4$^+$ T cells regulate the immune response in general, by influencing the antigen-processing of antigen-presenting cells. It now seems clear that the preferential induction of different subsets of CD4$^+$ T cells by intravenous versus subcutaneous route is not restricted to leishmanial antigens. Spleen cells from mice injected subcutaneously with sheep red blood cells produced substantially higher levels of IL-3 and IL-3 message compared to those from mice injected intravenously with the same antigen (Lelchuk et al. 1989).

7 Conclusion

The current working hypothesis regarding immune regulation in leishmaniasis can be summarised as follows. Infection of the mammalian host by promastigotes leads rapidly to the establishment of amastigotes in the macrophages. Depending on the genetic constitution of the host, this can lead either to limited multiplication of the parasites or to the uncontrolled replication of amastigotes. The former leads to the preferential induction of protective (CD4$^+$, T_{H1}-like) T cells whereas the latter activates the disease-promoting (CD4$^+$, T_{H2}-like) T cells. The two different subsets of CD4$^+$ T cells can also be induced by immunisation with killed parasites or soluble antigens by different routes of antigen administration. The intravenous/-intraperitoneal route preferentially induces the protective T cells whereas the subcutaneous/intramuscular route leads to the disease-promoting T cells. The precise mechanism of such preferential T-cell subset activation is unknown. It is likely that the two types of T cells recognise distinct epitopes being presented in a selective way by the antigen-presenting cells (APC). If this is true, and the determining factor is not the T-cell recognition repertoire but antigen epitope selection by APC, then identification of the host protective T_{H1} epitopes or presenting the otherwise disease-promoting T_{H2} epitopes in a manner to activate T_{H1} cells by appropriate adjuvants, a realistic and chemically defined vaccine may be developed.

The protective T cells secrete IFN-γ upon specific antigen stimulation. IFN-γ is a potent macrophage activator, and it induces macrophages to kill intracellular parasites. In contrast, the disease-promoting T cells can elaborate IL-3 and IL-4 which inhibit the activation of macrophages by IFN-γ. IL-3 is a multi-potent factor for the differentiation of haematopoietic progenitor cell and cells of the macrophage lineage. It may function by promoting macrophage differentiation without the accompanying activation. The mechanism by which IL-3 and IL-4 modulate the MAF activity of IFN-γ is at present unknown. It may be that they are able to down-regulate the IFN-γ receptor on macrophages, or alternatively they may function through internal signalling. This raises an intriguing question as to the possibility that the suppressor T-cell factors which were extensively described several years ago may indeed be some of the lymphokines discussed here.

The operational definition of immune suppression in leishmaniasis, in terms of abrogation of host-protective immunity of antigen-specific T_{H1} cells, can now be explained in terms of specific activation of a distinct subset of T_{H2} cells. The means by which this T_{H2} cell inhibits T_{H1}-cell function is emerging and appears to be via the arena of macrophages. Leishmaniasis therefore offers a convenient and biologically relevant model for the study of immune regulation, possibly leading to the detailed analysis of the mechanism of induction and interaction of subsets of T cells at the molecular level. This would have important implications in immunology in general and for the control of leishmaniasis in particular.

References

Arthur RP, Mason D (1986) T cells that help B cell responses to soluble antigen are distinguishable from those producing interleukin 2 on mitogenic or allogeneic stimulation. J Exp Med 163: 774–786

Behforouz NC, Wenger CD, Mathison BA (1986) Prophylactic treatment of BALB/c mice with cyclosporine A and its analog B-5-49 enhances resistance to *Leishmania major*. J Immunol 136: 3067–3075

Blackwell JM (1983) *Leishmania donovani* infection in heterozygous and recombinant H-2 haplotype mice. Immunogenetics 18: 101–109

Blackwell JM, Roberts MB, Alexander J (1985a) Response of BALB/c mice to leishmanial infection. Curr Top Microbiol Immunol 122: 97–106

Blackwell JM, Hale C, Roberts MB, Ulczak OM, Liew FY, Howard JG (1985b) An H-11-linked gene has a parallel effect on *Leishmania major* and *Leshmania donovani* infections in mice. Immunogenetics 21: 385–395

Bottomly K (1988) A functional dichotomy in $CD4^+$ T lymphocytes. Immunol Today 9: 268–274

Bradley DJ (1977) Regulation of *Leishmania* populations within the host. II. Genetic control of acute susceptibility of mice to *Leishmania donovani* infection. Clin Exp Immunol 30: 130–140

Button LL, McMaster WR (1988) Molecular cloning of the major surface antigen of *Leishmania*. J Exp Med 167: 724–729

Carvalho EM, Teixeira R, Johnson WD (1981) Cell-mediated immunity in American visceral leishmaniasis: reversible immunosuppression during acute infection. Infect Immun 33: 498–503

Cillari E, Liew FY, Lelchuk R (1986) Suppression of interleukin-2 production by macrophages in susceptible BALB/c mice infected with *Leishmania major*. Infect Immun 54: 386–394

Cillari E, Liew FY, LoCampo P, Milano S, Mansueto S, Salerno A (1988) Suppression of IL-2 production by cryopreserved peripheral blood mononuclear cells from patients with active visceral leishmaniasis in Sicily. J Immunol 140: 2721–2726

Crocker PR, Davies EV, Blackwell JM (1987) Variable expression of the murine natural resistance gene *Lsh* indifferent macrophage populations infected in vitro with *Leishmania donovani*. Parasite Immunol 9: 705–719

Greenblatt CL (1980) The present and future of vaccination for cutaneous Leishmaniasis. In: Mizrahi A, Hertman I, Klinberg MA (eds) New developments with human and veterinary vaccines. Liss, New York, p 259–285

Gorczynski RM (1985) Immunization of susceptible BALB/c mice against *Leishmania braziliensis*. II. Use of temperature-sensitive avirulent clones of parasite for vaccination purposes. Cell Immunol 94: 11–20

Gorczynski RM (1986) Do sugar residues contribute to the antigenic determinants responsbile for protection and/or abolition of protection in leishmania-infected BALB/c mice? J Immunol 137: 1010–1016

Haldar JP, Ghose S, Saha KC, Ghose AC (1983) Cell-mediated immune response in Indian kala-azar and post kala azar dermal leishmaniasis. Infect Immun 42: 702–709

Heinzel FP, Sadick MD, Holaday BJ, Coffman RL, Locksley RM (1989) Reciprocal expression of interferon-γ or interleukin 4 during the resolution or progression of murine leishmaniasis. Evidence for expansion of distinct helper T cell subsets. J Exp Med 169: 59–72

Herman R (1980) Cytophilic and opsonic antibodies in visceral leishmaniasis in mice. Infect Immun 28: 585–593

Ho M, Koech DK, Iha DM, Bryceson ADM (1983) Immunosuppression in Kenyan visceral leishmaniasis. Clin Exp Immunol 51: 207–214

Howard JG, Hale C, Liew FY (1980) Genetically determined susceptibility to *Leishmania tropica* infection is expressed by haematopoietic donor cells in mouse radiation chimaeras. Nature 288: 161–162

Howard JG, Hale C, Liew FY (1981) Immunological regulation of experimental cutaneous leishmaniasis. IV. Prophylactic effect of sublethal irradiation as a result of abrogation of suppressor T cell generation in mice genetically susceptible to *Leishmania tropica* infection. J Exp Med 153: 557–568

Howard JG, Nicklin S, Hale C, Liew FY (1982) Prophylactic immunisation against experimental leishmaniasis. I. Protection induced in mice genetically vulnerable to fatal *Leishmania tropica* infection. J Immunol 129: 2206–2211

Janeway CA (1975) Cellular cooperation during in vivo anti-hapten antibody response. I. The effect of cell number on the response. J Immunol 114: 1394–1401

Lelchuk R, Carrier M, Kahl L, Liew FY (1989) Distinct IL-3 activation profile induced by intravenous versus subcutaneous routes of immunisation. Cell Immunol 122: 338–349

Lelchuk R, Gravely R, Liew FY (1988) Susceptibility to murine cutaneous leishmaniasis correlates with the capacity to generate interleukin-3 in response to leishmania antigen in vitro. Cell Immunol 111: 66–76

Liew FY (1983) Specific suppression of responses to *Leishmania tropica* by a cloned T-cell line. Nature 305: 630–632

Liew FY (1986) Cell-mediated immunity in experimental cutaneous leishmaniasis. Parasitol Today 2: 260–270

Liew FY (1989) Functional heterogeneity of $CD4^+$ T cells in leishmaniasis. Immunol Today 10: 40–45

Liew FY, Dhaliwal JS (1987) Distinctive cellular immunity in genetically susceptible BALB/c mice recovered from *Leishmania major* infection or after subcutaneous immunisation with killed parasites. J Immunol 138: 4450–4456

Liew FY, Parish CR (1974) Lack of correlation between cell-mediated immunity to the carrier-hapten helper effect. J Exp Med 139: 779–784

Liew FY, Hale C, Howard JG (1982) Immunologic regulation of experimental cutaneous leishmaniasis. V. Characterisation of effector and specific suppressor T cells. J Immunol 128: 1917–1922

Liew FY, Howard JG, Hale C (1984) Prophylactic immunisation against experimental leishmaniasis. III. Protection against fatal *Leishmania tropica* infection induced by irradiated promastigotes involves $Lyt\text{-}1^+2^-$ T cells that do not mediate cutaneous DTH. J Immunol 132: 456–461

Liew FY, Millott S, Li Y, Lelchuk R, Chan WL, Ziltener H (1989) Macrophage activation by interferon-gamma from host-protective T-cells is inhibited by interleukin (IL) 3 and IL-4 produced by disease-promoting T-cells in Leishmaniasis. Eur J Immunol 19: 1227–1232

Liew FY, Singleton A, Cillari E, Howard JG (1985) Prophylactic immunisation against experimental leishmaniasis. V. Mechanism of anti-protective blocking effect induced by subcutaneous immunisation against *Leishmania major* infection. J Immunol 135: 2102–2107

Liew FY, Hodson K, Lelchuk R (1987) Prophylactic immunisation against experimental leishmaniasis. VI. Comparison of protective and disease-promoting T cells. J Immunol 139: 3112–3117

Louis JA, Mendonca S, Titus RG, Cerottini JC, Cerny A, Zinkernagel R, Milon G, Marchal G (1986) The role of specific T cell subpopulations in murine cutaneous leishmaniasis. In: Cinader B, Miller RG (eds) Progress in immunology. VI. Academic, New York, p 762–769

Marrack PC, Kappler JW (1975) Antigen-specific and non-specific mediators of T-cell/B-cell cooperation. I. Evidence for their production by different T-cells. J Immunol 114: 1116–1125

Maue J, Behin R (1982) Leishmaniasis. In: Cohen S, Warren KS (eds) Immunology of parasitic infections. Blackwell, p 299–335

Mitchell GF, Handman E (1985) T lymphocytes recognise *Leishmania* glycoconjugates. Parasitol Today 2: 61–63

Mitchell GF, Curtis JM, Scollay RG, Handman E (1981) Resistance and abrogation of resistance to cutaneous leishmaniasis in reconstituted BALB/c nude mice. Aust J Exp Biol Med Sci 59: 539–554

Modabber F (1987) The leishmaniasis. In: Maurice J, Pearce AM (eds) Tropical disease research, a global partnership, eighth programme report, TDR. World Health Organisation, Geneva, p 99–112

Morimoto C, Letvin NL, Distaso JA, Aldrich WR, Schlossman SF (1985) The isolation and characterisation of the human suppressor inducer T cell subset. J Immunol 134: 1508–1515

Mosmann TR, Coffman RL (1987) Two types of mouse helper T cell clone—implications for immune regulation. Immunol Today 8: 223–227

Mossmann TR, Cherwinski H, Bond MW, Giedlin MA, Coffman RL (1986) Two types of murine helper T cell clone. I. Definition according to profiles of lymphokine activities and secreted proteins. J Immunol 136: 2348–2357

Parish CR, Liew FY (1972) Immune response to chemically modified flagellin. III. Enhanced cell-mediated immunity during high and low gene antibody tolerance to flagellin. J Exp Med 135: 298–311

Pearson RD, Steigbigel RT (1980) Mechanism of lethal effect of human serum upon *Leishmania donovani*. J Immunol 125: 2195–2201

Petersen EA, Neva FA, Barral A, Correa-Coronas R, Bogaert-Diaz H, Martinex D, Ward FE (1984) Monocyte suppression of antigen-specific lymphocyte responses in diffuse cutaneous leishmaniasis patients from the Dominican Republic. J Immunol 132: 2603–2608

Powrie F, Mason D (1988) Phenotypic and functional heterogeneity of $CD4^+$ T cells. Immunol Today 9: 274–277

Preston PM, Dumonde DC (1976) Experimental cutaneous leishmaniasis. V. Protective immunity in subclinical and self-healing infection in the mouse. Clin Exp Immunol 23: 126–138

Preston PM, Carter RL, Leuchars E, Davies AJS, Dumonde DC (1972) Experimental cutaneous leishmaniasis. III. Effects of thymectomy on the course of infection of CBA mice with *Leishmania tropica*. Clin Exp Immunol 10: 337–357

Reiner NE, Finke JH (1983) Interleukin 2 deficiency in murine *Leishmania donovani* and its relationship to depressed spleen cell responses to phytohemagglutinin. J Immunol 131: 1487–1491

Rezai HR, Ardekali SM, Amirhakimi G, Kharazmi A (1978) Immunological features of kala-azar. Am J Trop Med Hyg 27: 1079–1082

Rezai HR, Farrell J, Soulsby El (1980) Immunological responses of *L. donovani* infection in mice and significance of T cell in resistance to experimental leishmaniasis. Clin Exp Immunol 40: 508–514

Russell DG, Alexander J (1988) Effective immunization against cutaneous leishmaniasis with defined membrane-antigens reconstituted into liposomes. J Immunol 140: 1274–1279

Sacks DL, Scott PA, Asofsky R, Sher FA (1984) Cutaneous leishmaniasis in anti-IgM-treated mice: enhanced resistance due to functional depletion of a B cell-dependent T cell involved in the suppressor pathway. J Immunol 132: 2072–2077

Sadick MD, Locksley RM, Tubbs C, Raff HV (1986) Murine cutaneous leishmaniasis: resistance correlates with the capacity to generate interferon-γ in response to leishmania antigens in vitro. J Immunol 136: 655–661

Scott PA, Farrell JP (1981) Experimental cutaneous leishmaniasis. I. Nonspecific immunosuppression in BALB/c mice infected with *Leishmania tropica*. J Immunol 127: 2395–2400

Scott P, Natovitz P, Sher A (1986) B lymphocytes are required for the generation of T cells that mediate healing of cutaneous leishmaniasis. J Immunol 137: 1017-1021

Scott P, Pearce E, Natovitz P, Sher A (1987) Vaccination against cutaneous leishmaniasis in a murine model. I. Induction of protective immunity with a soluble extract of promastigotes. J Immunol 139: 221–227

Scott P, Natovitz P, Coffman RL, Pearce E, Sher A (1988a) Immunoregulation of cutaneous leishmaniasis. T cell lines that transfer protective immunity or exacerbation belong to different T helper subsets and respond to distinct parasite antigens. J Exp Med 168: 1675–1684

Scott P, Pearce E, Natovitz P, Sher A (1988b) Adoptive transfer of protective immunity against lethal *Leishmania major* infection with an L3T4 (Th1) T cell clone recognising a low molecular weight parasite antigen. FASEB J 2: A1256

Silver J, Benacerraf B (1974) Dissociation of T cell helper function and delayed hypersensitivity. J Immunol 113: 1872–1875

Solbach W, Forberg K, Kammerer E, Bogdan C, Rollinghoff M (1986) Suppressive effect of cyclosporin A on the development of *Leishmania tropica*-induced lesions in genetically susceptible BALB/c mice J. Immunol 137:702–707

Sterm JJ, Oca MJ, Rublin BY, Anderson SL, Murray HW (1988) Role of L3T4$^+$ and Lyt-2$^+$ cells in experimental visceral leishmaniasis. J Immunol 140: 3971–3977

Titus RG, Lima GC, Engers HD, Louis JA (1984) Exacerbation of murine cutaneous leishmaniasis by adoptive transfer of parasite-specific helper T cell populations capable of mediating *Leishmania major*-specific delayed-type hypersensitivity. J Immunol 133: 1594–1600

Titus RG, Ceredig R, Cerottini JC, Louis JA (1985) Therapeutic effect of anti-L3T4 monoclonal antibody GK 1.5 on cutaneous leishmaniasis in genetically susceptible BALB/c mice. J Immunol 135: 2108-2114

Titus RG, Milon G, Marchal G, Vassalli P, Cerottini J-C, Louis J (1987) Involvement of specific Lyt-2$^+$ T cells in the immunological control of experimentally induced murine cutaneous leishmaniasis. Eur J Immunol 17: 1429–1433

Titus R, Kinsey P, Thoedos C, Louis J (1988) Induction of resistance to experimental cutaneous leishmaniasis in genetically-susceptible BALB/c mice by immunisation with chemically-mutagenised non-infective clones of *Leishmania major*. FASEB J 2: A887

Wallis AE, McMaster WR (1987) Identification of *Leishmania* Genes encoding proteins containing tandemly repeating peptides. J Exp Med 166: 724–729

T-Cell Antigens and Epitopes in Malaria Vaccine Design

M. F. GOOD[1] and L. H. MILLER[2]

1 Introduction

T cells are central to the development of an immune response, whether it be a humoral or a cell-mediated response. In this sense, all protein antigens can be regarded as potential T-cell antigens. Recent developments in understanding the processes involved in T-cell activation now allow us rigorously to examine the T-cell response to a given organism in terms of antigen specificity, epitope identification, the effects of antigenic variation, the role of different T-cell subsets in immunity to different pathogens, etc. In terms of vaccine development, such a rigorous approach has not been previously used, as empirical measures have often sufficed. However, the development of vaccines for complex organisms, for example, the malaria parasite, may require more insight from a molecular immunological approach. This will certainly be the case if one hopes to develop a "subunit" vaccine consisting of one or a few antigens or parts of them. In this review, the T-cell response to already identified malaria vaccine candidate antigens is examined, the role of cellular immunity to malaria is discussed and the problem of identifying other important antigens with respect to T-cell activation is addressed.

Malaria is initiated with the bite of an infectious mosquito. Sporozoites are inoculated by the mosquito and are then subsequently cleared by various organs, with those going to the liver developing further into merozoites and eventually emerging from hepatocytes (after about 1 week in the case of *Plasmodium falciparum*) ready to invade red blood cells. It is this phase in the red blood cells which is responsible for the morbidity and mortality of malaria. Eventually, sexual forms develop in the red blood cells—the male and female gametocytes—which are taken up by the mosquito during its blood meal. These gametocytes, which are inside red blood cells and thus not susceptible to antibody attack, emerge from the red blood cells in the mosquito midgut and fertilize, giving rise to zygotes, then ookinetes, and eventually sporozoites.

In terms of vaccine development, present strategies are to develop vaccines against each stage in the life cycle. This is sensible since malaria immunity is stage

[1] The Tropical Health Program, Queensland Institute of Medical Research, Bramston Terrace, Herston 4006, Queensland, Australia

[2] The Laboratory of Parasitic Diseases, National Institute of Allergy and Infectious Diseases, National Institutes of Health, Bethesda MD 20892, USA

Current Topics in Microbiology and Immunology, Vol. 155

specific. In general terms, a sporozoite vaccine would aim to block sporozoites before they invaded hepatocytes or to kill infected hepatocytes; a blood-stage vaccine would aim to block merozoite invasion of red blood cells or to destroy infected erythrocytes or the parasites inside infected erythrocytes; and a sexual-stage vaccine (transmission-blocking vaccine) would aim to kill gametocytes prior to uptake by mosquitoes or to block gamete fertilization or zygote development in the mosquito midgut.

From a philosophical point of view, the difficulties with developing a malaria vaccine relate to our poor understanding of the state of natural immunity to malaria. Adults living in a malaria-endemic region often have detectable levels of parasites in their blood, and many individuals may have parasite levels that are below detection. These people are rarely sick from the malaria parasites they harbor. In contrast, people with no previous exposure to malaria (e.g., young children in Africa) can become quite ill with high parasitemia. The immune adult also differs from the nonimmune in that symptoms caused by equivalent levels of parasitemia are greater in the nonimmune. This "tolerance" to malaria is well described (CLARK 1987). A malaria vaccine that converts the immune status of child into that of an immune adult in terms of suppressing parasitemia may leave the vaccinee quite prone to symptomatic attacks of malaria—unless such a vaccine can provide sterile (complete) immunity. A nonsterilizing vaccine may nevertheless limit parasitemia to such an extent to prevent the lethal consequences of falciparum malaria. The problem is thus obvious. To provide sterile immunity, a vaccine will have to induce better immunity than the natural infection can (supernatural immunity). Furthermore, because of the difficulties of revaccinating individuals in developing countries, it will have to do so following a single immunization.

Philosophically, therefore, there are two approaches to malaria vaccine development. The first is to understand natural immunity and develop a vaccine that may result in some morbidity but hopefully reduced mortality. The second approach would be to design a vaccine that, following a single dose, will give long-lasting sterile "supernatural" immunity. Both approaches merit consideration.

2 Sporozoite Immunity

A sporozoite vaccine will have to induce sterile immunity to be effective. This is because sporozoite immunity is stage specific, and any parasites that escaped surveillance during the sporozoite or liver stage would not be susceptible during the blood stage. There is little evidence to support the view that a vaccine that blocked most, but not all, sporozoites would allow the subsequent malaria infection to be less severe.

In laboratory animals it is possible successfully to immunize with irradiated sporozoites. This immunity is mediated by T cells (CHEN et al. 1977) of which cytotoxic T-lymphocytes (CTL) appear to be the most important (SCHOFIELD et al. 1987; WEISS et al. 1988) and to be antibody specific for the circumsporozoite (CS) protein (POTOCNJAK et al. 1980). Unfortunately, it is seldom possible to immunize humans with sporozoites (CLYDE et al. 1973; RIECKMAN et al. 1979; HOFFMAN et al. 1987), probably due to immunity-induced variation within the T-cell epitopes of the CS and possibly other sporozoite or liver stage proteins (see below). Here, thus, is an example where it may be necessary to develop a vaccine inducing "supernatural" immunity.

Early in this decade it was shown that monoclonal antibodies specific for the CS protein of a murine malaria could passively transfer protection to a naive mouse (POTOCNJAK et al. 1980). Sera from sporozoite-immunized mice, however, do not transfer protection even though the donor mice are themselves protected (SPITANLY et al. 1976; EGAN et al. 1987). Similarly, humans who have circulating antisporozoite antibodies from natural exposure to sporozoites are not protected (HOFFMAN et al. 1987). One goal, then, is to develop a vaccine that both quantitatively and qualitatively is more immunogenic than sporozoites themselves. The use of different adjuvants, lymphokines, coupling procedures, or conformationally restricted peptides may be important considerations. In a murine vaccine trial, it has been shown that the method of coupling the B epitope to the carrier protein is critical in achieving an immunogen that can generate protective antibodies (ZAVALA et al. 1987).

2.1 The T-Cell Response to the CS Protein

The CS protein covers malaria sporozoites and binds the majority of antisporozoite antibodies. In fact, almost all these antibodies bind to the central repetitive segment of the protein. This protein initially created excitement when it was observed that CS-specific monoclonal antibodies could passively transfer protection in a murine system (POTOCNJAK et al. 1980). Vaccine development was then aimed at developing an immunogen that could induce a high-titer anti-CS antibody response. The T-cell response was originally examined to determine the immunogenicity of a subunit vaccine derived from the central repetitive epitope of the CS protein, $(NANP)_n$. Two groups independently reported that the central repeats of the CS protein of *P. falciparum* were poorly immunogenic to mice, and that only mice bearing the $I\text{-}A^b$ allele responded to $(NANP)_n$ in terms of T-cell proliferation or antibody production following immunization without a carrier protein (GOOD et al. 1986; DEL GIUDICE et al. 1986; TOGNA et al. 1986). The results suggested that such a vaccine in humans would be poorly immunogenic, and that natural boosting following sporozoite exposure would not occur. The results of human vaccine studies (BALLOU et al. 1987; HERRINGTON et al. 1987) as well as studies looking at the T-cell response to the CS repeats of humans living in endemic regions (GOOD et al. 1988b) have validated the predictions although other factors may have also contributed to the poor immunogenicity in the human vaccine studies.

These results prompted us to examine the immunogenicity of the entire CS protein. Using either a recombinant vaccinia virus containing the CS gene or purified recombinant CS protein, different H-2 congenic mice were immunized, and the antibody response was determined (GOOD et al. 1987; DONTFRAID et al. 1989). H-

2^b and H-2^k mice were high responders to the CS protein of *P. falciparum* whereas other strains were low responders or in some cases (H-2^r, H-2^q, for example) nonresponders. The T-cell response to the repeats appeared to explain why the H-2^b mice were high responders, but H-2^k mice were unable to respond to the repeats. The epitope on the CS protein that they were responding to was predicted by an alogorithm and verified (GOOD et al. 1987). It was located on the carboxylterminal side of the repeats. Soon thereafter, it was realized that this region was one of the few regions of variation in the entire protein (DE LA CRUZ et al. 1987).

Studies in humans from endemic regions using overlapping peptides spanning the entire CS protein then identified this as well as two other variant regions as the immunodominant human T-cell epitopes for the protein. The overabundance of nonsynonymous (coding change) mutations in the CS protein led DE LA CRUZ and his colleagues (1987) to postulate that pressure at the protein level was responsible for the mutations in the protein. The overlap of the human T-cell epitopes with the variant regions suggested that this pressure was immune pressure from T cells (GOOD et al. 1988b). Since T cells do not recognize native protein but only epitopes in association with products of the major histocompatibility complex (MHC), the pressure must have occurred during a cellular stage in the life cycle of the parasite. The obvious conclusion was that it was occurring during the hepatocyte stage following sporozoite invasion. The identified epitopes were, however, recognized by proliferating and the helper T cells (CD4) and as such would have been MHC class II associated. Since hepatocytes do not bear such molecules (at least to the level of detection), the hypothesis was difficult to reconcile. However the identification of CD8 cells as being the major effector cells in sporozoite immunity (SCHOFIELD et al. 1987; WEISS et al. 1988), the subsequent identification of CS-specific CTL following sporozoite immunization, and the localization of a CD8 epitope to the variant region of the protein (KUMAR et al. 1988) suggested that the immune pressure selecting variation in the CS protein was from CTL. The overlap of the CD4 epitopes with the variable region was then easily explained by the known similarities of CD4 and CD8 epitopes (BERZOFSKY et al. 1987; MARYANSKI et al. 1986; TOWNSEND et al. 1986).

Thus, although a given minimal CD4 epitope may well not be a CD8 epitope in a given individual, the similar physicochemical properties of both types of epitopes often results in similar regions of proteins being immunogenic for both sets of T cells. However, it is well to include a few caveats to the above hypothesis. If hepatocytes do bear class II molecules (below detection), or if such molecules are induced during sporozoite invasion and the subsequent immune response, selection could occur directly via CD4 lymphocytes. Alternatively, even though the vast majority of antisporozoite antibodies (ZAVALA et al. 1983) are specific for the central repeats, the variation in the nonrepeat region could theoretically be selected by antibodies directed to this region. Such antibodies have not been identified, but antibodies that can block sporozoite invasion in vitro (ALEY et al. 1986) do bind near a smaller variable domain at the aminoterminal side of the repeats, and it has been suggested that the variation here was selected by antibody (DE LA CRUZ et al. 1987). This region, although recognized by murine T cells, was not an immunodominant T-cell epitope in one endemic population of humans from West Africa (GOOD et al. 1988b).

The hypothesis outlined above requires demonstration that induction of CTL to a particular CS epitope leads to protection. It has been demonstrated in the mouse model following immunization with a CS-recombinant salmonella that CS-specific T cells, in the absence of antibody, can protect (SADOFF et al. 1988), and passive transfer of CS-specific CTL clones can protect in the mouse (ROMERO et al. 1989).

The observed variation within the CS protein would appear to hinder the development of a CS-based vaccine designed to stimulate protective T cells. Indeed, the variation in the CS protein often precludes recognition by T cells stimulated by a different variant (DE LA CRUZ et al. 1988; DE GROOT et al. submitted). More recently, however, SINIGAGLIA and colleagues have reported that nonimmune as well as immune T cells from individuals of diverse HLA types respond by proliferation to a sequence corresponding to a conserved region of the CS protein, with the exception that two cysteine residues were replaced by alanine residues (SINIGAGLIA et al. 1988a, b). Some of the T-cell clones were able to respond to CS protein extracted from sporozoites. This sequence, if it could stimulate helper T cells, could be very useful for an antibody-based vaccine.

A vaccine designed to stimulate cellular immunity would not have to rely solely on CS-specific immunity. Theoretically, any antigen expressed in the liver which was immunogenic for CTL, and which was invariant would suffice. Other hepatic-stage antigens have been identified (GUERIN-MARCHAND et al. 1987; SZARFMAN et al. 1988) but their ability to stimulate CTL has not been addressed. Clearly, however, if variation within the CS protein can be selected by CTL, variation within other proteins could also be selected by CTL, providing the proteins were not functional proteins with obvious constraints upon their ability to vary. Although it is important to search for such proteins, our enthusiasm is somewhat tempered by the observation by HOFFMAN and colleagues (1987) that natural sporozoite immunity among endemic populations rarely occurs. In terms of future directions, the most sensible route may be to attempt to design a vaccine inducing "supernatural" CS-specific humoral immunity. Although natural boosting of antibody levels by sporozoites may be unattainable in many people, it may be possible to maintain antibodies of sufficient quality and quantity for prolonged periods of time following primary vaccination. While such a vaccine, if developed, may be suitable for tourists, it should only be used cautiously as the sole means of malaria prevention for endemic populations. The potential risk would be that if and when such induced immunity waned, there would be no backup blood-stage immunity, and severe malaria might ensue.

3 Blood-Stage Immunity

T cells play an important role in blood-stage immunity and will play a major role in any asexual vaccine. Whether the primary mechanism of immunity is cellular or antibody mediated, there is the need for CD4 T-cell memory. There is, of course, evidence for the requirement of both limbs of the immune response. Certainly, there is accumulating evidence of the great importance of cellular immunity in protection from malaria in different host species. In murine and avian malarias, naturally acquired immunity to different species of *Plasmodium* can develop in animals devoid of B cells or circulating antibodies (FERRIS et al. 1973; RANK and WEIDANZ 1976; GRUN and WEIDANZ 1981, 1983). In contrast, passive transfer of large quantities of immune sera is unable to protect nude mice at all against the lethal *P. vinckei* (KUMAR et al. 1989). However, in *P. yoelii*, it has been demonstrated that antibodies against the major merozoite surface antigen (MSA-1, see below) can transfer protection to mice (MARJARIAN et al. 1984). In many mouse malarias, however, μ-suppressed mice can be immunized by repeated infection and cure (for example, GRUN and WEIDANZ 1983; KUMAR et al. 1989). In vaccine trials in monkeys it has been demonstrated that animals can be protected in the absence of antibodies that block parasite invasion into red cells (MILLER et al. 1977; BUTCHER et al. 1978). In Sudan, an association has been observed between clinical immunity to *P. falciparum* and a nonantibody serum factor capable of causing intraerythrocytic parasite death or "crisis" (JENSEN et al. 1983). "Crisis" has been associated with a cellular immune response to malaria and the subsequent liberation of lymphokines. In contrast, however, in a region of Indonesia studied by the same group, immunity appeared to be based mainly on antimerozoite antibodies (JENSEN et al. 1984).

Recently, a CD4 T-cell clone was developed from a mouse that was immunized by infection and cure, which could passively protect nude mice from *P. chabaudi* (BRAKE et al. 1988). Identifying the antigen responsible for stimulating the T clone will be an important step in development of a vaccine for stimulating cellular immunity. Possible methods include the screening of expression libraries with T-cell clones (MUSTAFA et al. 1988) or probing immunoblotted antigen with T-cell lines or clones ("T-cell Western;" LAMB and YOUNG 1987). It could be inferred from this elegant experiment (BRAKE et al. 1988) that a single T site on a single malaria antigen should be able to stimulate cellular immunity and lead to protection. At this point, however, that has not been demonstrated. However, stimulation of a population of memory T cells may not be enough in itself for success. The role of T cells in protection from malaria probably relates to their ability to activate a population of monocytes which can mediate intracellular parasite death via the further liberation of monokines and oxygen free radicals (CLARK and HUNT 1983; DOCKRELL and PLAYFAIR 1983; TAVERNE et al. 1987; CLARK et al. 1987). This scenario probably occurs in the spleen where parasites are filtered through a network of T cells, B cells, and monocytes. Splenic architecture appears to be critical in this process (L. WEISS et al. 1986). Splenectomy, followed by reconstitution of splenic cells results in total loss of naturally acquired immunity (OSTER et al. 1980; GRUN et al. 1985; KUMAR et al. 1989).

In relevance to this discussion, transfer of immune T cells can restore immunity to an immunized but T-cell depleted animal providing that the animal is eusplenic (KUMAR et al. 1989). Thus, a vaccine capable of stimulating cellular immunity alone may be ineffective if the vaccine cannot correctly modify splenic architecture. Although a CD4 T-cell clone could transfer protection against *P. chabaudi* to naive mice, the animals developed a significant parasitemia following challenge. This could possibly be related to an unprepared splenic architecture. Certain vaccine vectors (e.g., salmonella, bacille Calmette-Guérin) can certainly modify splenic architecture, but the question remains whether this modification is suitable to allow malaria-immune T cells to operate effectively. Only vaccine trials with recombinant vectors will answer this question.

If suitable antigens can be identified, problems of nonresponsiveness and genetic restriction may be major problems. Identification of a number of different antigens, each of which can be protective in a "responder" individual will be necessary. A cocktail vaccine combining all such antigens in a suitable recombinant vector will probably be necessary.

Antibody certainly plays a role in protection. Early experiments in children with acute *P. falciparum* malaria who received γ-globulin from immune adults demonstrated that peripheral parasitemias declined significantly (Cohen et al. 1961). Curiously, there was a 3-day delay before the decline in parasitemia. The possibility cannot be excluded that antibody was enhancing antigen presentation to T cells, as has been described for the mouse (Ron and Sprent 1987). This is a role for antibody in protection that has not seriously been considered, but that may be very important. There is more convincing evidence from monkey malarias of the direct role of antibody. In monkeys immunized with the 140-kDa proteins of *P. knowlesi* and challenged, the initial parasitemia reaches a certain level before immunity comes in and drives down the parasitemia (Klotz et al. 1987). Eventually, however, mutants arise that lack expression of this merozoite surface protein. Thus there is selection for rare mutants. When the same monkeys are reinfected, again the wild parasites grow to a parasitemia of about 1% before immune mechanisms come into play and select for rare mutants.

From a humoral vaccine development aspect, the two most studied, falciparum blood-stage antigens are the Pf155/RESA antigen of ring-infected erythrocytes (Perlman et al. 1984; Coppel et al. 1984) and Pf195 or MSA-1 antigen from the surface of merozoties (Holder and Freeman 1981; Holder et al. 1985; Hall et al. 1984). Both of these antigens, or fragments from them, have been used in vaccine studies with variable success (Hall et al. 1984; Perrin et al. 1984; Siddiqui et al. 1987; Collins et al. 1986; Patarroyo et al. 1987, 1988). Pf155/RESA initially created excitement when it was demonstrated that antibodies directed against it could inhibit merozoite invasion in vitro. Like most malaria antigens, Pf155/RESA contains repetitive and nonrepetitive regions. By contrast with the T epitopes from the CS protein, the repetitive constant region of the protein appears to be the most immunodominant, although the nonrepetitive flanking regions are also seen by T cells from humans living in endemic regions (Kabilan et al. 1988; Rzepczyk et al. 1988). T cells from nonexposed as well as exposed humans respond to peptides from this protein. When used in a vaccine study in monkeys, 9 of 14 animals were protected, but some of the "protected" animals nevertheless developed high parasitemias (0.1%–3.7%) (Collins et al. 1986). Correlations between degree of protection and merozoite invasion inhibition by serum antibodies or T-cell stimulation were not examined, so it is not clear what the principal mode of protection was in this study.

In similar studies using MSA-1, six of six Africans with a history of malaria exposure, as well as four of four Europeans with no history of malaria exposure or serum MSA-1 specific antibodies responded to synthetic peptides mimicking the native protein (SINIGAGLIA et al. 1988c). Unlike the human response to the CS protein, the individuals responded to a conserved region of the protein. It would seem unlikely that such T cells would be protective in the four Europeans with no history of exposure. MSA-1 specific antibody may play a role in protection, however. This antigen has also shown promise in vaccine studies in monkeys (PERRIN et al. 1984; HALL et al. 1984; SIDDIQUI et al. 1987). In one study (SIDDIQUI et al. 1987) three of three monkeys showed complete protection (no peripheral parasitemia) following challenge. Unfortunately, the mechanism of protection (humoral versus cellular) was not examined in any study. It has, however, been demonstrated that immunization can lead to protection following heterologous challenge (HALL et al. 1984), even though the protein is known to be polymorphic (WEBER et al. 1986; TANABE et al. 1987), suggesting that the conserved region of the protein may stimulate protective immunity. By contrast, in the most promising human vaccine trial to date, PATTAROYO et al. (1988) constructed a synthetic peptide vaccine containing MSA-1 specific sequences and could find no correlation between protection and either humoral or cellular immune responses.

An inherent difficulty with vaccine studies is that the number of presently identified antigens is very limited. Clearly, if an antigen has been identified, and antibodies against it can block parasite development in vitro, it would seem reasonable to assess its capacity as a vaccine. The critical factor in the success of the vaccine trial then relates back to the method of identification of the antigen: was it identified by differential screening with immune versus nonimmune sera, for example, or by another method thought to have predictive value? The problem here is that we do not know enough about the immunobiology of the parasite to rely with confidence on any method of antigen identification for vaccine design. One solution is to make no presumptions about the vaccine potential of any antigen and to select antigens virtually at random. However, the lack of availability of large numbers of monkeys makes such a route impractical for falciparum vaccine studies. These types of studies are feasible in the mouse, however, where large numbers of recombinant antigens from a murine malaria library could be tested. Homologous antigens could then be identified from a falciparum library.

4 Transmission-Blocking Immunity

T cells appear to play a major role in the development of or failure to develop immunity to the sexual stages of malaria. Such immunity is mediated by a T-cell dependent antibody response and by cellular mechanisms. The antigens recognized by protective antibodies are the gamete or zygote surface antigens (CARTER et al. 1984). Antibodies either prevent gamete fertilization or block zygote development in the gut of the mosquito after being taken up with gametocytes during a blood meal. The antigens which form the targets of these antibodies have molecular masses of

230 kDa, 48/45 kDa, 40 kDa, and 25 kDa. The 25-kDa antigens, unlike the others, appears to be expressed mainly on the zygotes, but not on the gametocytes (in the human host). The other antigens are expressed both on the mosquito and human stages.

Although antibodies can block transmission, sera from most humans living in endemic regions contain undetectable levels of antibodies to any of the known transmission-blocking target antigens of *P. falciparum* (GRAVES et al. 1988; CARTER et al. 1988; QUAKYI et al. 1989), and about one-half of falciparum gametocyte carriers are infectious to mosquitoes (GRAVES et al. 1988). However, there may be more naturally occurring transmission-blocking immunity to *P. vivax* (DE ZOYSA et al. 1988). The epidemic curves for vivax malaria can be adequately explained only based on the occurrence of transmission-blocking immunity modifying the full impact of transmission.

In the case of falciparum, only 20%–40% of humans appear capable of responding to the 230-kDa antigen, fewer than 10% can respond to that of the 48/45 or 40 kDa, and no sera contain antibodies to the 25-kDa antigen (see below). This lack of response to the antigens of 230 kDa, 48/45 kDa, and 40 kDa does not appear to be related to individual differences in exposure to malaria or to gametocytes in particular since all individuals in one study responded to crude blood-stage antigen, and very few of those who responded to the 230-kDa antigen responded to other gamete surface antigens (CARTER et al. 1988; QUAKYI et al. 1989). Studies using these antigens in H-2 congenic mice suggest that nonresponsiveness is *Ir* gene-controlled (GOOD et al. 1988a). Following immunization with cloned zygotes, two of six strains of H-2 congenic mice responded to the 230-kDa antigen, a different two strains responded to the 48/45-kDa antigen, and a single strain responded to the 40-kDa antigen. Why, then, are neither humans nor mice good responders to these gamete antigens? The murine data would suggest that there is a limited number of functional T-helper epitopes on these antigens. Perhaps, in a similar fashion to the CS protein, the parasite has evolved such that these antigens contain fewer T-helper epitopes and as such are less immunogenic. Such a strategy would confer a survival advantage on the parasite.

The 25-kDa zygote surface antigen differs in expression and immunogenicity from the 230-kDa, 48/45-kDa, and 40-kDa antigens. It is probably expressed only in the mosquito midgut and not in the human host. The evidence is as follows. In the avian malaria, *P. gallinaceum*, which has a highly homologous protein, the protein is not expressed in the chicken and is first seen after zygote formation (CARTER and KAUSHAL 1984). A rodent malaria, *P. berghei* also only appears to express the protein after gametogenesis in the mosquito midgut (WINGER et al. 1988). It is difficult to know whether the falciparum protein is expressed in humans since any in vitro manipulation could lead to transformation from gametocytes to gametes (the mosquito stage). The actual test is to immunize with the 25-kDa antigen and then see whether there is boosting following natural infection. Human sera from falciparum endemic regions does not contain anti-25-kDa antibodies, probably because humans are not exposed to this antigen. In contrast, all H-2 congenic mouse strains immunized with zygotes (which express the protein) generate anti-25-kDa antibodies (GOOD et al. 1988a) suggesting that the protein would be immunogenic in humans if they were exposed to it (recent data suggests that humans and mice respond to similar T epitopes; DONTFRAID et al. 1989). The 25-kDa parasite protein that is not exposed to immune pressure from the human host would not need to evolve evasion mechanisms such as a poorly immunogenic molecule or epitope variation. In fact, following the recent cloning of this protein (KASLOW et al. 1988), the subsequent search for variation revealed a single nucleotide substitution among eight geographically distinct isolates (KASLOW et al. 1989).

The lack of variation in the 25-kDa protein makes it a promising candidate for a transmission-blocking vaccine. However, the lack of expression in humans indicates that natural boosting of the immune response by the parasite will not occur. In combination with other measures of malaria control, however, such a vaccine could have a significant effect. A 25-kDa vaccine could be either a recombinant 25-kDa protein or merely a synthetic peptide containing a blocking epitope (if a linear blocking epitope can be found on the protein) joined to a carrier. A blocking monoclonal antibody has been generated against this protein (VERMEULEN et al. 1985), and an epitope identified (VAN AMERONGEN et al. 1989). A subunit vaccine containing a transmission-blocking epitope (B epitope) joined to a carrier offers the advantage of avoiding possible autoimmune complications. Like many malaria proteins (MCLAUGHLIN et al. 1987), the 25-kDa protein contains segments which are homologous to human sequences (KASLOW et al. 1988). The epidermal growth factor (EGF)-like domains of the 25-kDa protein could stimulate antibodies against host proteins which contain these domains, for example, the low-density lipoprotein receptor (SUDHOF et al. 1985). Providing that this domain on the 25-kDa protein was not part of the blocking epitope, it may be wise to omit it from a vaccine.

A little-studied area of transmission-blocking immunity is the role of cellular immunity. There has been one report that immune $CD4^+$ T cells, upon adoptive transfer, can block transmission of malaria to the mosquito (HARTE et al. 1985). Such T cells are probably effective in the host, rather than the vector, and may kill intracellular gametocytes via a similar mechanism to which immune $CD4^+$ T cells can kill intracellular asexual-stage parasites. Since CD4 effector mechanisms against infected red cells that express no MHC class II are probably nonspecific, why is the killing selectively against gametocytes and no asexual parasites? One possible explanation is greater susceptibility of gametocytes to nonspecific mediators.

Vaccination with dead parasites and subunits has led to protection of varying degrees in experimental malarias, and it should be possible to replicate this in humans. However, one must take into consideration the findings on variation and low immunogenicity in vaccine design. Problems with variation may have been less prevalent in the experimental systems since the parasite is often passaged in nonimmune animals. Multivalent vaccines and the correct adjuvants may help to overcome the problem in the human situation, but the use of an attenuated vaccine (WAKI et al. 1983) should not be ignored in spite of obvious problems of safety and parasite culture. While not suitable for the sporozoite or transmission-blocking vaccines, they may have a definite role in blood-stage protection.

References

Aley SB, Bates MD, Tam JP, Hollingdale MR (1986) Synthetic peptides from the circumsporozoite proteins of *Plasmodium falciparum* and *Plasmodium knowlesi* recognize the human hepatoma cell line Hep G2-A16 in vitro. J Exp Med 164: 1915–1922

Ballou WR, Hoffman SL, Sherwood JA, Hollingdale MR, Neva FA, Hockmeyer WT et al. (1987) Safety and efficacy of a recombinant DNA *Plasmodium falciparum* sporozoite vaccine. Lancet: 1277–1281

Berzofsky JA, Cease KB, Cornette JL, Spouge JL, Margalit H, Berkower IJ, Good MF, Miller LH, DeLisi C (1987) Protein antigenic structures recognized by T cells: potential applications to vaccine design. Immunol Rev 98: 9–52

Brake DA, Long CA, Weidanz WP (1988) Adoptive protection against *Plasmodium chabaudi adami* malaria in athymic nude mice by a cloned T cell line. J Immunol 140: 1989–1993

Butcher GA, Mitchell GH, Cohen S (1978) Antibody mediated mechanisms of immunity to malaria induced by vaccination with *Plasmodium knowlesi* merozoites. Immunology 34: 77–86

Carter R, Kaushal DC (1984) Characterization of antigens on mosquito midgut stages of *Plasmodium gallinaceum*. III. Changes in zygote surface proteins during transformation to mature ookinetes. Mol Biochem Parasitol 13: 235–241

Carter R, Miller LH, Rener J, Kaushal DC, Kumar N, Graves PM, Grotendorst CA, Gwadz RW, French C, Wirth D (1984) Target antigens in malaria transmission blocking immunity. Philos Trans R Soc Lond [Biol] 307: 201–213

Carter R, Graves PM, Quakyi IA, Good MF (1989) Restricted or absent immune responses in human populations to *Plasmodium falciparum* gamete antigens which are targets of malaria transmission-blocking antibodies. J Exp Med 169: 135–147

Chen DH, Tigelaar RE, Weinbaum FI (1977) Immunity to sporozoite-induced malaria infection in mice. I. The effect of immunization of T and B cell-deficient mice. J Immunol 118: 1322-1327

Clark A (1987) Monokines and Lymphokines in malarial pathology. Ann Trop Med Parasitol 81: 577–585

Clark IA, Hunt NH (1983) Evidence for reactive oxygen intermediates causing hemolysis and parasite death in malaria. Infect Immun 39: 1–6

Clark IA, Hunt NH, Butcher GA, Cowden WB (1987) Inhibition of murine malaria (*Plasmodium chabaudi*) in vivo by recombinant interferon-γ or tumor necrosis factor and its enhancement by butylated hydroxyanisole. J Immunol 139: 3493–3496

Clyde DF, Most H, McCarthy VC, Vanderberg JP (1973) Immunization of man against sporozoite-induced falciparum malaria. Am J Med Sci 266: 169–177

Cohen S, McGregor IA, Carrington S (1961) Gamma-globulin and acquired immunity to human malaria. Nature 192: 733–737

Collins WE, Anders RF, Pappaioanou M, Campbell GH, Brown GV, Kemp DJ, Coppel RL, Skinner JC, Andrysiak PM, Favaloro JM, Corcoran LM, Broderson JR, Mitchell GF, Campbell CC (1986) Immunization of *Aotus* monkeys with recombinant proteins of an erythrocyte surface antigen of *Plasmodium falciparum*. Nature 323: 259–262

Coppel RL, Cowman AF, Anders RF, Bianco AE, Saint RB, Lingelbach KR, Kemp DJ, Brown GV (1984) Immune sera recognise on erythrocytes a *Plasmodium falciparum* antigen composed of repeated amino acid sequences. Nature 310: 789–792

de la Cruz VF, Lal AA, McCutchan TF (1987) Sequence variation in putative functional domains of the circumsporozoite protein of *Plasmodium falciparum*: implications for vaccine development. J Biol Chem 262: 11935–11939

de la Cruz VF, Maloy WL, Miller LH, Lal AA, Good MF, McCutchan TF (1988) Lack of cross-reactivity between variant T cell determinants from malaria circumsporozoite protein. J Immunol 141: 2456–2460

Del Giudice G, Cooper JA, Merino J, Verdini AS, Pessi A, Togna AR, Engers HD, Corradin G, Lambert P-H (1986) The antibody response in mice to carrier-free synthetic polymers of *Plasmodium falciparum* circumsporozoite repetitive epitope is I-A^b-restricted: possible implications for malaria vaccines. J Immunol 137: 2952–2955

de Zoysa APK, Herath PRJ, Abhayawardana TA, Padmalal UKGK, Mendis KN (1988) Modulation of human malaria transmission by anti-gamate transmission blocking immunity. Trans R Soc Trop Med Hyg 82: 548–553

Dockrell HM, Playfair JHL (1983) Killing of blood stage malaria parasites by hydrogen peroxide. Infect Immun 39: 456–459

Dontfraid F, Cochran MA, Pombo D, Knell JD, Quakyi IA, Kumar S, Houghten RA, Berzofsky JA, Miller LH, Good MF (1989) Human and murine CD4 T-cell epitopes map to the same region of the malaria circumsporozoite protein: limited immunogenicity of sporozoites and circumsporozoite protein. Mol Biol Med 5: 185–196

Ferris DH, Beamer PD, Stutz DR (1973) Observations on the response of dysgammaglobulinemic chickens to malarial infection. Avian Dis 17: 12

Good MF, Berzofsky JA, Maloy WL, Hayashi Y, Fujii N, Hockmeyer WT, Miller LH (1986) Genetic control of the immune response in mice to a *Plasmodium falciparum* sporozoite vaccine. Widespread nonresponsiveness to single malaria T epitope in highly repetitive vaccine. J Exp Med 164: 655–660

Good MF, Maloy WL, Lunde MN, Margalit H, Cornette JL, Smith GL, Moss B, Miller LH, Berzofsky JA (1987) Construction of synthetic immunogen: use of new T helper epitope on malaria circumsporozoite protein. Science 235: 1059–1062

Good MF, Miller LH, Kumar S, Quakyi IA, Keister D, Adams JH, Moss B, Berzofsky JA, Carter R (1988a) Limited immunological recognition of critical malaria vaccine candidate antigens. Science 242: 574–577

Good MF, Pombo D, Quakyi IA, Riley EM, Houghten RA, Menon, Alling DW, Berzofsky JA, Miller LH (1988b) Human T cell recognition of the circumsporozoite protein of *Plasmodium falciparum.* Immunodominant T cell domains map to the polymorphic regions of the molecule. Proc Natl Acad Sci USA 85: 1199–1203

Graves PM, Carter R, Burkot TR, Quakyi IA, Kumar N (1988) Antibodies to *Plasmodium falciparum* gamete surface antigens in Papua New Guinea sera. Parasite Immunol 10: 209–218

Grun JL, Weidanz WP (1981) Immunity to *Plasmodium chabaudi adami* in the B-cell deficient mouse. Nature 290: 143–145

Grun JL, Weidanz WP (1983) Antibody-dependent immunity to reinfection malaria in B-cell deficient mice. Infect Immun 41: 1197–1204

Grun JL, Long CA, Weidanz WP (1985) Effects of splenectomy on antibody-independent immunity to *Plasmodium chabaudi adami* malaria. Infect Immun 48: 853–858

Guerin-Marchand C, Druihle P, Galey B, Londono A, Patarapotikul J, Beaudoin RL, Dubeaux C, Tartar A, Mercereau-Puijalon O, Langsley G (1987) A liver-stage-specific antigen of *Plasmodium falciparum* characterized by gene cloning. Nature 329: 164–167

Hall R, Hyde JE, Goman M, Simmons DL, Hope IA, Mackay M, Scaife J (1984) Major surface antigen gene of a human malaria parasite cloned and expressed in bacteria. Nature 311: 379–382

Harte PG, Rogers NC, Targett GAT (1985) Role of T cells in preventing transmission of rodent malaria. Immunology 56: 1–7

Herrington DA, Clyde DF, Losonsky G, Cortesia M, Murphy FR, Davis J et al. (1987) Safety and immunogenicity in man of a synthetic peptide malaria vaccine against *Plasmodium falciparum* sporozoites. Nature 328: 257–259

Hoffman SL, Oster CN, Plowe CV, Woollett GR, Beier JC, Chulay JD et al. (1987) Naturally acquired antibodies to sporozoites do not prevent malaria: vaccine development implications. Science 237: 639–649

Holder AA, Freeman RR (1981) Biosynthesis and processing of a *Plasmodium falciparum* schizont antigen recognized by immune serum and a monoclonal antibody. J Exp med 156: 1528–1538

Holder AA, Lockyer MJ, Odink KG, Sandhu JS, Riveros-Moreno V, Nicholls SC, Hillman Y, Davey LS, Tizard MLV, Svhwarz RT, Freeman RR (1985) Primary structure of the precursor to the three major surface antigens of *Plasmodium falciparum* merozoites. Nature 317: 270–273

Jensen JB, Boland MT, Allan JS, Carlin JM, Vande Waa JA, Divo AA, Akood MAS (1983) Association between human serum-induced crisis forms in cultured *Plasmodium falciparum* and clinical immunity to malaria in Sudan. Infect Immun 41: 1302–1311

Jensen JB, Hoffman SL, Boland MT, Akood MAS, Laughlin LW, Kurniawan L, Marwoto HA (1984) Comparison of immunity to malaria in Sudan and Indonesia: crisis-form versus merozoite-invasion inhibition. Proc Natl Acad Sci USA 81: 922–925

Kabilan L, Troye-Blomberg M, Perlmann H, Andersson G, Hogh B, Petersen E, Bjorkman A, Perlmann P (1988) T-cell epitopes in Pf155/RESA, a major candidate for a *Plasmodium falciparum* malaria vaccine. Proc Natl Acad Sci USA 85: 5659–5663

Kaslow DC, Quakyi IA, Syin C, Raum MG, Keister DB, Coligan JE, McCutchan TF, Miller LH (1988) A vaccine candidate from the sexual stage of human malaria that contains EGF-like domains. Nature 333: 74-76

Kaslow DC, Quakyi IA, Keister DB (1989) Minimal variation in a vaccine candidate from the sexual stage of *Plasmodium falciparum.* Mol Biochem Parasitol 32: 101–104

Klotz FW, Hudson DE, Coon HG, Miller LH (1987) Vaccination-induced variation in the 140 kD merozoite surface antigen of *Plasmodium knowlesi* malaria. J Exp Med 165: 359–367

Kumar S, Miller LH, Quakyi IA, Keister DB, Houghten RA, Maloy WL, Moss B, Berzofsky JA, Good MF (1988) Cytotoxic T cells specific for the circumsporozoite protein of *Plasmodium falciparum*. Nature 334: 258–260

Kumar S, Good MF, Dontfraid F, Vinetz JM, Miller LH (1989) Interdependence of $CD4^+$ T cells and malarial spleen in immunity to *Plasmodium vinckei vinckei*. Relevance to vaccine development. J Immunol 143: 2017–2023

Lamb JR, Young DB (1987) A novel approach to the identification of T-cell epitopes in *Mycobacterium tuberulosis* using human T-lymphocyte clones. Immunology 60: 1–5

Marjarian WR, Daly TM, Weidanz WP, Long CA (1984) Passive immunization against murine malaria with an IgG3 monoclonal antibody. J Immunol 132: 3131–3137

Maryanski JL, Pala P, Corradin G, Jordan BR, Cerottini J-C (1986) H-2-restricted cytolytic cells specific for HLA can recognize a synthetic HLA peptide. Nature 324: 578–579

McLaughlin GL, Benedik MJ, Campbell GH (1987) Repeated immunogenic amino acid sequences of *Plasmodium* species share sequence homologies with proteins from humans and human viruses. Am J Trop Med Hyg 37: 258–262

Miller LH, Powers KG, Shiroishi T (1977) *Plasmodium knowlesi:* functional immunity and antimerozoite antibodies in *Rhesus* monkeys after repeated infection. Exp Parasitol 41: 105–111

Mustafa AS, Oftung F, Deggerdal A, Gill HK, Young RA, Godal T (1988) Gene isolation with human T lymphocyte probes. Isolation of a gene that expresses an epitope recognized by T cells specific for *Mycobacterium bovis* BCG and pathogenic mycobacteria. J Immunol 141: 2729–2733

Oster CN, Koontz LC, Wyler DJ (1980) Malaria in asplenic mice: effects of splenectomy, congenital asplenia, and splenic reconstitution on the course of infection. Am J Trop Med Hyg 29: 1138–1142

Patarroyo ME, Romero P, Torres ML, Clavijo P, Moreno A, Martinez A, Rodriguez R, Guzman F, Cabezas E (1987) Induction of protective immunity against experimental infection with malaria using synthetic peptides. Nature 328: 629–632

Patarroyo ME, Amador R, Clavijo P, Moreno A, Guzman F, Romero P, Tascon R, Franco A, Murillo LA, Ponton G, Trujillo G (1988) A synthetic vaccine protects humans against challenge with asexual blood stages of *Plasmodium falciparum* malaria. Nature 332: 158–161

Perlman H, Berzins K, Wahlgren M, Carlsson J, Bjorkman A, Patarroyo ME, Perlman P (1984) Antibodies in malarial sera to parasite antigens in the membrane of erythrocytes infected with early asexual stages of *Plasmodium falciparum*. J Exp Med 159: 1686–1704

Perrin LH, Merkli B, Loche M, Chizzolini C, Smart J, Richle R (1984) Antimalarial immunity in saimiri monkeys. Immunization with surface components of asexual blood stages. J Exp Med 160: 441–451

Potocnjak P, Yoshida N, Nussenzweig RS, Nussenzweig V (1980) Monovalent fragments (Fab) of monoclonal antibodies to a sporozoite surface antigen (Pb44) protect mice against malaria infection. J Exp Med 151: 1504–1513

Quakyi IA, Otoo LN, Pombo D, Sugars LY, Menon A, Riley EM, DeGroot AS, Johnson A, Alling D, Miller LH, Good MF (1989) Differential nonresponsiveness in humans of candidate *Plasmodium falciparum* vaccine antigens. Am J Trop Med Hyg (in press)

Rank RG, Weidanz WP (1976) Nonsterilizing immunity in avian malaria: an antibody-independent phenomenon. Proc Soc Exp Biol Med 151: 257–259

Rieckmann KH, Beaudoin RL, Cassells JS, Sell KW (1979) Use of attenuated sporozoites in the immunization of human volunteers against falciparum malaria. Bull WHO57 [Supp 1]: 261–265

Romero P, Maryanski JL, Corradin G, Nussenzweig RS, Nussenzweig V, Zavala F (1989) Cloned cytotoxic T cells recognize an epitope in the circumsporozoite protein and protect against malaria. Nature 341: 323–326

Ron Y, Sprent J (1987) T cell priming in vivo: a major role for B cells in presenting antigen to T cells in lymph nodes. J immunol 138: 2848–2856

Rzepczyk CM, Ramasamy R, Ho PC-L, Mutch DA, Anderson KL, Duggelby RG, Doran TJ, Murray BJ, Irving DO, Woodrow GC, Parkinson D, Brabin BJ, Alpers MP (1988) Identification of T epitopes within a potential *Plasmodium falciparum* vaccine antigen. A study of human lymphocyte responses to repeat and nonrepeat regions of Pf155/RESA. J Immunol 141: 3197–3202

Sadoff JC, Ballou WR, Baron LS, Majarian WR, Brey RN, Hockmeyer WT, Young JF, Cryz SJ, Ou J, Lowell GH, Chulay JD (1988) Oral *Salmonella typhimurium* vaccine expressing circumsporozoite protein protects against malaria. Science 240: 336–338

Schofield L, Villaquiran J, Ferreira A, Schellekens H, Nussenzweig RS, Nussenzweig V (1987) Gamma interferon, CD8 T cells and antibodies required for immunity to malaria sporozoites. Nature 330: 664–666

Siddiqui WA, Tam LQ, Kramer KJ, Hui GSN, Case SE, Yamaga KM, Chang SP, Chan EBT, Kan S-C (1987) Merozoite surface coat precursor protein completely protects *Aotus* monkeys against

Plasmodium falciparum malaria. Proc Natl Acad Sci USA 84: 3014–3018
Sinigaglia F, Guttinger M, Gillessen D, Doran DM, Takacs B, Matile H, Trzeciak A, Pink JRL (1988a) Epitopes recognized by human T lymphocytes on malaria circumsporozoite protein. Eur J Immunol 18: 633–636
Sinigaglia F, Guttinger M, Kilgus J, Doran DM, Matile H, Etlinger H, Trzeciak A, Gillessen D, Pink JRL (1988b) A malaria T-cell epitope recognized in association with most mouse and human MHC class II molecules. Nature 336: 778–780
Sinigaglia F, Takacs B, Jacot H, Matile H, Pink JRL, Crisanti A, Bujard H (1988c) Nonpolymorphic regions of p190, a protein of the *Plasmodium falciparum* erythrocytic stage, contain both T and B cell epitopes. J Immunol 140: 3568–3572
Spitalny GL, Rivera-Oritz C-I, Nussenzweig RS (1976) *Plasmodium berghei*: the spleen in sporozoite-induced immunity to mouse malaria. Exp Parasitol 40: 179–188
Sudhof TC, Goldstein JL, Brown MS, Russell DW (1985) The LDL receptor gene: a mosaic of exons shared with different proteins. Science 228: 815–822
Szarfman A, Walliker D, McBride JS, Lyon JA, Quakyi IA, Carter R (1988) Allelic forms of gp195, a major blood-stage antigen of *Plasmodium falciparum*, are expressed in liver stages. J Exp Med 167: 231–236
Tanabe K, Mackay M, Goman M, Scaife JG (1987) Allelic dimorphism in a surface antigen gene of the malaria parasite *Plasmodium falciparum*. J Mol Biol 195: 273–287
Taverne J, Tavernier J, Fiers W, Playfair JHL (1987) Recombinant tumor necrosis factor inhibits malaria parasites in vivo but not in vitro. Clin Exp Immunol 67: 1–4
Togna AR, Del Guidice G, Verdini AS, Bonelli F, Pessi A, Engers HD, Corradin G (1986) Synthetic *P. falciparum* circumsporozoite peptides elicit heterogeneous $L3T4^+$ T cell proliferative responses in $H\text{-}2^b$ mice. J Immunol 137: 2956–2960
Townsend ARM, Rothbard J, Gotch FM, Bahadur G, Wraith D, McMichael AJ (1986) The epitopes of influenza nucleoprotein recognized by cytotoxic T lymphocytes can be defined with short synthetic peptides. Cell 44: 959–968
Van Amerongen A, Sauerwein RW, Beckers PJA, Meloen RH, Meuwissen JHET (1989) Identification of a peptide sequence of the 25 kD surface protein of *Plasmodium falciparum* recognized by transmission-blocking monoclonal antibodies: implications for synthetic vaccine development. Parasite Immunol 11: 425–428
Vermeulen AN, Ponnudurai T, Beckers PJA, Verhave J-P, Smits MA, Meuwissen JHET (1985) Sequential expression of antigens on sexual stages of *Plasmodium falciparum* accessible to transmission-blocking antibodies in the mosquito. J Exp Med 162: 1460–1476
Waki S, Yonome I, Suzuki M (1983) *Plasmodium falciparum*: attenuation by irradiation. Exp Parasitol 56: 339-345
Weber JL, Leininger WM, Lyon JA (1986) Variation in the gene encoding a major merozoite surface antigen of the human malaria parasite *Plasmodium falciparum*. Nucleic Acids Res 14: 3311–3323
Weiss L, Geduldig U, Weidanz W (1986) Mechanisms of splenic control of murine malaria: reticular cell activation and the development of a blood-spleen barrier. Am J Anat 176: 251–285
Weiss WR, Sedegah M, Beaudoin RL, Miller LH, Good MF (1988) $CD8^+$ T cells (cytotoxic/suppressors) are required for protection in mice immunized with malaria sporozoites. Proc Natl Acad Sci USA 85: 573–576
Winger LA, Tirawanchai N, Nicholas J, Carter HE, Smith JE, Sinden RE (1988) Ookinete antigens of *Plasmodium berghei*. Appearance on the zygote surface of an M_r 21 kD determinant identified by transmission-blocking monoclonal antibodies. Parasite Immunol 10: 193–207
Zavala F, Cochrane AH, Nardin EH, Nussenzweig RS, Nussenzweig V (1983) Circumsporozoite proteins of malaria parasites contain a single immunodominant region with two or more identical epitopes. J Exp Med 157: 1947–1957
Zavala F, Tam JP, Barr PJ, Romero PJ, Ley V, Nussenzweig RS, Nussenzweig V (1987) Synthetic peptide vaccine confers protection against murine malaria. J Exp Med 166: 1591–1596

Cytotoxic T Cells in Immunity to *Theileria parva* in Cattle

W. I. Morrison and B. M. Goddeeris

1 Introduction

Theileria are tick-borne protozoan parasites which in their mammalian hosts successively utilise leukocytes and erythrocytes for completion of their life cycle. The parasites are found predominantly in ruminants. In domestic cattle, there are two species, namely *T. annulata* and *T. parva*, which cause economically important diseases. *T. parva* occurs throughout a large part of East and Central Africa where it causes an acute, usually fatal disease known as East Coast fever (ECF) (W.I. Morrison et al. 1986; Irvin and Morrison 1987). Control of the disease relies largely on regular application of acaricides to prevent tick infestation. This practice is costly, time consuming and can lead to selection of acaricide-resistant ticks. Thus an effective method of imunising against the disease would have a major impact on cattle production in ECF-endemic areas. To this end, studies have been undertaken to define the host immune responses involved in immunity against *T. parva* with the aim of identifying protentially protective antigens. These studies have yielded evidence that major histocompatibility complex (MHC) restricted cytotoxic T cells are important in mediating immunity.

In this paper, we review current information on *T. parva*-specific cytotoxic T cell responses and, in particular, focus on the role of the MHC in determining the parasite strain specificity of the responses.

2 The Host-Parasite Relationship

2.1 The parasite life cycle

Infection of cattle with *T. parva* is initiated when sporozoites, deposited by the tick vector during feeding, gain entry into lymphocytes. This occurs by receptor-mediated endocytosis, and during the subsequent 12–24 h the host cell membrane

* B.M.G. is supported by the AGCD/ABOS (General Administration for Development Cooperation) of Belgium. This is ILRAD publication number 728
International Laboratory for Research on Animal Diseases, P.O. Box 30709, Nairobi, Kenya

Current Topics in Microbiology and Immunology, Vol. 155

surrounding the parasite is destroyed so that the parasite comes to lie free in the cytoplasm (Fawcett et al. 1984). Within 24–48 h of invading a lymphocyte, the sporozoite starts to develop to a multinucleate body, termed a schizont. This is associated with activation of the host cell which begins to proliferate. At each cell division, the parasite also divides so that both daughter cells are infected (Hulliger et al. 1964). Thus the infection is established and becomes disseminated by clonal expansion of the small population of lymphocytes initially infected by the parasite. Later in the infection, schizonts undergo merogony, and merozoites thus formed infect erythrocytes, giving rise to prioplasms which are infective for the tick.

Susceptible cattle usually die within 4 weeks of infection with the parasite. In such animals, large numbers of parasitised lymphoid cells are found throughout the lymphoid system and are associated with extensive lymphocytolysis (Morrison et al. 1981; Irvin and Morrison 1987). Parasitised cells also invade non-lymphoid tissues, particularly the lungs and gastrointestinal tract and, in the lungs, commonly result in severe pulmonary oedema. Thus, it is the schizont stage of the parasite which is responsible for most of the pathology of the disease.

The relationship of the parasite with the host cells enables parasitised cells to grow continuously in culture; parasitised cell lines can be established either by culturing cells from infected cattle or by infecting normal lymphocytes in vitro with sporozoites (Brown et al. 1973; Brown 1983). The latter culture system has proved extremely useful for experiments to identify the host cell types infected with *T. parva* and for studies of T-cell responses to the parasite.

2.2 Host Cell Types Infected by the Parasite

The production in the past few years of monoclonal antibodies (MAb) specific for different populations of bovine lymphocytes and accessory cells has made it possible to define which cell types are infected with *T. parva*. The susceptibility of different populations of cells to infection and transformation by the parasite in vitro has been tested by incubating cells purified with a fluorescence-activated cell sorter, with suspensions of *T. parva* sporozoites, and subsequently monitoring the establishment of cell lines following distribution of the cells at limiting dilution in the wells of microtitre plates (Baldwin et al. 1988). These experiments showed that B-lymphocytes, both major subpopulations of T-lymphocytes (BoT4$^+$ and BoT8$^+$) and an additional population of lymphocytes lacking B-cell and T-cell markers could readily be infected and establish cell lines. Purified monocytes and granulocytes did not give rise to cell lines. However, when unfractionated populations of peripheral blood mononuclear cells (PBM) were infected with the parasite, the cell lines which established invariably had the phenotype of T cells. Moreover, phenotypic analyses of infected cells in cattle undergoing lethal infections with *T. parva* have demonstrated that the majority of infected cells in vivo are T-lymphocytes (Emery et al. 1988). These findings indicated that while all of the presently defined subpopulations of lymphocytes are susceptible to infection with *T. parva*, T-lymphocytes dominate the infections in vivo.

2.3 Properties of Parasitised Cells

The growth characteristics of *Theileria*-infected lymphocytes are similar to those of neoplastically transformed cells. This apparent transformed state is dependent on the continued presence of the parasite, as the removal of parasites by specific drug treatment causes cells to revert to a non-proliferative state (PINDER et al. 1981). Constitutive production, by infected cells, of a growth factor with functional properties and apparent molecular weight similar to those of interleukin 2 (IL-2) has been demonstrated (BROWN and LOGAN 1986) and suggested as an important contributory factor to maintenance of growth of infected cells. These experiments were conducted with a BoT8^{+} T-cell clone which was infected in vitro with *T. parva* and prior to infection did not produce the growth factor. Experiments carried out by DOBBELAERE et al. (1988) have also demonstrated that recombinant human IL-2 supports and potentiates the growth of infected cells when they are cultured at low cell densities. While these observations indicate that an autocrine mechanism of production and consumption of growth factors may contribute to the growth of infected cells, they do not shed light on the primary events within the cell which lead to the transformed state. Nevertheless, the observation that infected cells produce and are responsive to growth factors has potentially important implications in the pathogenesis and immunology of the disease. Thus, on the one hand, functional changes induced in host lymphocytes by the parasite might influence the generation of parasite-specific immune responses and, on the other, soluble mediators elaborated during the induction of such immune responses may modulate the growth or behaviour of the parasitised cells.

3 Immunity Against *T. parva*

3.1 Immunisation of Cattle

Cattle can be immunised against *T. parva* by inoculating them with a potentially lethal dose of sporozoites followed by treating them for several days with the antibiotic oxytetracycline (NEITZ 1953; RADLEY et al. 1975a, d). This regimen results in a transient mild infection from which the animals recover and are subsequently immune to challenge with the same parasite. Attempts to immunise cattle with non-viable parasite antigens have generally been unsuccessful (reviewed in MORRISON et al. 1986).

3.2 Parasite Strain Heterogeneity

A shortcoming of the infection and treatment immunisation procedure which has limited its practical application is that immunisation with one stock of the parasite does not provide protection against all other stocks (Radley et al. 1975b, c; Irvin et al. 1983). However, parasite strain heterogeneity is probably limited as the use of mixtures of two or three stocks for immunisation has provided protection against experimental challenge with a number of stocks isolated in different geographical locations and against field challenge (Irvin 1985). The precise immunological characterisation of parasite stocks is complicated by the fact that in cross-protection experiments, breakthrough infections usually do not occur reciprocally between parasite stocks. Thus, there are many examples of a parasite stock that protects against another stock but not vice versa. Moreover, when breakthrough infections occur, they often do so only in a proportion of animals. These findings may be due in part to the fact that the parasite stocks are uncloned and therefore may be heterogeneous mixtures. Support for this notion comes from recent studies with parasite-specific MAbs and DNA probes. DNA sequences present as multiple copies in the *Theileria* genome have been cloned and, when used as probes on Southern blots of DNA prepared from different parasite stocks, detect restriction fragment length polymorphism (Conrad et al. 1987). These probes also detect differences in the DNA from parasites within cloned cell lines derived from the same parasite stock (P.A. Conrad et al., in press). Similar differences between and within parasite stocks have been observed with MAbs specific for a parasite antigen which shows marked polymorphism among populations of *T. parva* (Shapiro et al. 1987; B.M. Goddeeris and P.G. Toye, unpublished data). It is likely that genetic recombination between parasite populations contributes to these phenotypic and genotypic differences. Such recombination is well documented in other protozoan parasites such as malaria (Walliker et al. 1987) and trypanosomes (Jenni et al. 1986), and in *Theileria* there is morphological evidence of zygote formation from gametes during development in the tick (Melhorn and Schein 1976; Schein et al. 1977). In order to elucidate this question and to provide defined parasites for further immunological studies, efforts are currently being devoted to obtaining cloned populations of *Theileria* parasites.

3.3 Mechanisms of Immunity

Although cattle repeatedly exposed to sporozoites produce antibodies which, in vitro, neutralise the infectivity of sporozoites (Musoke et al. 1982), only a minor anti-sporozoite response is detected after a single immunisation by infection and treatment. In animals immunised in this way the protective immune responses are believed to be directed against schizont-infected lymphocytes (reviewed in W.I. Morrison et al. 1986). This is based on the observations that schizont-infected cells are often transiently detectable 7–9 days after challenge of immune cattle with sporozoites, and that cattle can be immunised with large numbers of viable schizont-infected cells, i.e. in the absence of exposure to sporozoites.

Given that the schizont stage of the parasite remains in an intracellular location during replication, it is difficult to envisage antibodies being effective against this stage of the parasite. Indeed, although immunisation results in readily detectable anti-schizont antibody responses, there is no evidence that such antibodies play a role in protection. Nor is there any evidence that cattle produce antibodies to parasite-specific antigens on the surface of infected cells (Creemers 1982). By inference, therefore, it would seem that immunity is likely to involve cell-mediated immune responses. This is supported by the findings that transfer of thoracic duct lymphocytes from immune to naive chimaeric twin calves protected against concurrent challenge with *T. parva* (Emery 1981) whereas attempts to transfer immunity with serum from immune cattle were unsuccessful (Muhammed et al. 1975).

4 *Theileria*-Specific T-Cell Responses

4.1 Cytotoxic T-Cell Responses

The first direct evidence that infections with *T. parva* induce cell-mediated immune responses was derived from experiments in which cattle were infected or immunised with the parasite and their PBM monitored for cytotoxic activity on parasitised cell lines. In cattle undergoing lethal infections, cytotoxic cells capable of killing allogeneic infected cells as well as murine YAC-1 cells were detected in the peripheral blood during the later stages of the infection (Emery et al. 1981). Somewhat surprisingly, these effectors did not kill autologous infected cells. The absence of killing of autologous cells may have been due to the presence of infected cells in the effector population which might act as cold target inhibitors of any effectors specific for autologous cells. At any rate, the cytotoxic cells detected clearly do not recognise target molecules on autologous cells. The identity of these effector cells and their target antigen specificity have not been investigated further.

By contrast to findings in cattle undergoing lethal infections, immunisation or challenge of cattle with *T. parva* results in the induction of cytotoxic T cells specific for parasitised lymphoblasts. These cytotoxic cells are transiently detectable in the peripheral blood at the time of remission of infection (Eugui and Emery 1981; Emery et al. 1981). They kill autologous parasitised cells but not uninfected lymphoblasts or cells from unrelated cattle infected with the same parasite. By selecting panels of target cells of defined MHC phenotypes and by testing the capacity of MAb specific for class I or class II MHC molecules to inhibit cytotoxicity, the cytotoxic cells were shown to be restricted by class I MHC determinants (Morrison et al. 1987b). In the majority of animals, there was a marked bias in the restriction of the cytotoxic T-cell response to one or other of the MHC haplotypes (all animals were heterozygous). Moreover, with the class I specificities represented, responses restricted by some specificities (or haplotypes) consistently predominated over responses restricted by others (Morrison et al. 1987b). The results indicated that there is a hierarchy in dominance among the class I MHC molecules that restrict the response. Subsequent studies of the effectors following stimulation in vitro demonstrated that they are T-lymphocytes belonging to the T8 subset (Goddeeris et al. 1986a).

The temporal relationship of the cytotoxic T-cell response with disappearance of parasitised cells in cattle undergoing challenge with *T. parva* indicates that the response may be important in control of the infection. Moreover, such a mechanism of immunity is compatible with the finding that establishment of infection in the animal is required for immunity to develop because of the need for T cells to recognise antigenic changes on the cell surface in the context of self MHC molecules.

To date the parasite-induced antigens recognised by the cytotoxic T cells have not been identified. In one instance, an apparently parasite-specific cell surface antigen was detected with a MAb (Newson et al. 1986); however when the parasitised cells were cloned and used to infect an allogeneic animal, infected cells isolated from the recipient animal did not express the antigen. In retrospect, with the information which has recently emerged on how viral antigens are presented to class I restricted T cells as small processed peptides on the surface of infected cells (Townsend et al. 1986), it is not surprising that a parasite-specific cell surface antigen could not be detected with antibodies.

4.2 Helper T-Cell Responses

The evaluation of non-cytotoxic T-cell responses against *Theileria*-infected cells has been difficult because of the fact that, in in vitro proliferative assays, parasitised cells induce proliferative responses of similar magnitude and kinetics in PBM from immune or naive cattle (Pearson et al. 1979; Goddeeris and Morrison 1987). However, experiments in which lymphocyte cultures were restimulated at weekly intervals in vitro with autologous parasitised cells showed that proliferative cultures of T cells from immune cattle could be maintained for 1–3 months, whereas similar cultures from naive cattle often showed a gradual diminution of proliferative activity (Goddeeris et al. 1986a). A large proportion of the proliferating cells from immune cattle were $BoT4^+$ $BoT8^-$ T-lymphocytes. Cloned populations of these cells were obtained and were shown to be specific for parasitised cells and restricted by class II MHC determinants (Baldwin et al. 1987). These cloned population had properties characteristic of helper T cells in that they proliferated, upon antigenic stimulation, in the absence of exogenous growth factors and were shown to produce T-cell growth factor activity.

In studies of murine and human T-cell responses, the observation that class I-restricted cytotoxic T cells grown in vitro usually require exogenous growth factors for maintenance of proliferation has led to the prevailing belief that class II restricted helper T cells are required for the generation of a cytotoxic T-cell response. However recent experiments carried out in mice (Heeg et al. 1987a, b) have demonstrated the existence of a population of $Ly2^+$ ($T8^+$) T cells which produce IL-2 following antigenic stimulation. Moreover, several studies in vivo in mice have shown that generation of virus-specific cytotoxic T-cell responses (Buller et al. 1987) and graft versus host and graft rejection responses (Sprent et al. 1986) can be mediated by $Ly2^+$ T cells in the absence of $L3T4^+$ ($T4^+$) T cells. In view of these findings, the role of $BoT4^+$ T cells in providing help in the generation of class I restricted cytotoxic T cells specific for *Theileria*-infected cells must remain speculative.

4.3 Parasite Strain Specificity of the Cytotoxic T-Cell Responses

Since the immunity induced by one stock of *T. parva* often does not provide protection against challenge with all other stocks of the parasite, one would expect to observe a degree of strain specificity in the protective immune responses. To address this question, the parasite strain specificity of *Theileria*-specific cytotoxic T-cell responses in cattle immunised with *T. parva* (Muguga), has been analysed on target cell lines infected with the Muguga and Marikebuni stocks. These two stocks are immunologically different in that cattle immunised with Marikebuni are immune to challenge with Muguga, whereas a proportion of animals immunised with Muguga are susceptible to challenge with Marikebuni (Irvin et al. 1983). In order to preclude the argument that differences in cytotoxicity might be due to the two parasites infecting different cell types, cloned T cells infected with the two parasites were prepared as target cells for most of the animals. In most instances, these cell lines were also cloned after infection to ensure that they did not contain mixed parasite populations.

The results from six cattle, three of which were reported on previously (Morrison et al. 1987b), are shown in Table 1. Cytotoxic cells generated in two of the animals were completely specific for Muguga-infected target cells, whereas effector cells from the remaining four cattle showed killing of target cells infected with either Muguga or Marikebuni parasites. Although these particular animals have not been challenged with the Marikebuni stock to determine whether the specificity of the response correlates with protection, the results clearly demonstrate

Table 1. Parasite strain specificity of the *Theileria*-specific cytotoxic T-cell response in six immune cattle challenged with *T. parva* (Muguga)

Donor of effector cells	Target cell line	BoLA phenotype[a]	Percent cytotoxicity on targets infected with[b]	
			T. parva (Muguga)	*T. parva* (Marikebuni)
B641	B641	w10/KN18	41	2
	T11.49(B641)[c]	w10/KN18	36	0
	B171	w7/KN18	59	0
C447	T16.13(C447)[c]	w7/w10	63	4
	C167	w4/w10	42	1
C234	C234	w6/w10	42	23
	C165	w6/w7	31	13
	T3.5(C196)[c]	w6/w7	44	2
C196	T3.5(C196)[c]	w6/w7	52	15
	C165	w6/w7	35	25
	C234	w6/w10	82	61
D247	D247	w6.2/w7	56	59
	D232	w6.2/w2	34	31
	T19.4(C887)[c]	w6.2/w10	47	37
D409	D409	w7/w10	65	73
	D247	w6.2/w7	43	76

[a] Cattle and parasitised cell lines were typed serologically for class I antigens as described by Teale et al. (1983)
[b] Results obtained at an effector to target ratio of 40:1 in a 4-h ^{51}Cr-release assay are presented.
[c] T-cell clone infected with *T. parva*.

that, as with protection, there is considerable heterogeneity in the specificity of the cytotoxic T-cell response among individual animals immunised with the same parasite stock.

5 Analyses with Cytotoxic T-Cell Clones

5.1 Generation of Cytotoxic T Cells In Vitro

The use of effector cells generated in vivo to analyse the antigenic relationship of different parasites is limited because of the likelihood that such populations contain cells with different antigenic specificites. Moreover, the levels of cytotoxicity detected in PBM of cattle undergoing immunisation or challenge with *T. parva* are often low and are detectable only for a few days. Therefore, for further studies of the antigenic specificity of the cytotoxic T cells, it was necessary to culture the effector cells in vitro and to obtain cloned populations. Details of the techniques used are described elsewhere (GODDEERIS and MORRISON 1988a).

Cultures containing *T. parva*-specific cytotoxic T cells are readily generated in vitro from PBM of immunised animals by repeated stimulation with autologous infected cells on a weekly basis. As with the in vivo response, the effector cells have been shown to be MHC class I restricted and are within the $BoT8^+$ T-cell subset (GODDEERIS et al. 1986a). In general the MHC restriction and strain specificity of these cultures are similar to those observed in vivo. In only one of eight cattle in which both the responses in vivo and in vitro were analysed was the MHC restriction of the effectors generated in vitro different from that of the in vivo effectors. In this case, there was evidence that this was due to a decrease in the level of expression of one of the MHC class I antigens on the infected cell line used to stimulate the culture.

Cytotoxic T-cell clones were derived from these cultures following removal of the $BoT4^+$ lymphocytes, which usually constituted over 60% of the cells, by complement-mediated lysis with a BoT4-specific MAb (GODDEERIS et al. 1986b). These clones showed potent killing activity (Fig. 1), giving maximum cytotoxicity at effector to target ratios of between 1:1 and 4:1. Schizonts were apparently released intact; however, since this stage of the parasite has a very poor capacity to infect lymphocytes, killing of the infected cell essentially eliminates the parasite.

5.2 Influence of the Immunising Parasite on Strain Specificity of the Cytotoxic T Cells

Cytotoxic T-cell clones generated from cattle immunised with the Muguga stock of *T. parva* varied in their parasite strain specificity. In some instances they killed

▶

Fig. 1a, b. Electron micrographs showing loose binding of a cytotoxic T-cell (*T*) to a parasitised lymphoblast observed 30 min after mixing the two populations (**a**) and lysis of a parasitised cell by a cytotoxic T-cell (*T*) observed 60 min after mixing the two populations (**b**). In each instance, the schizont is indicated with an *arrow*. Ultrastructural studies of the cells were carried out by Dr. S. Ito. (× 6000)

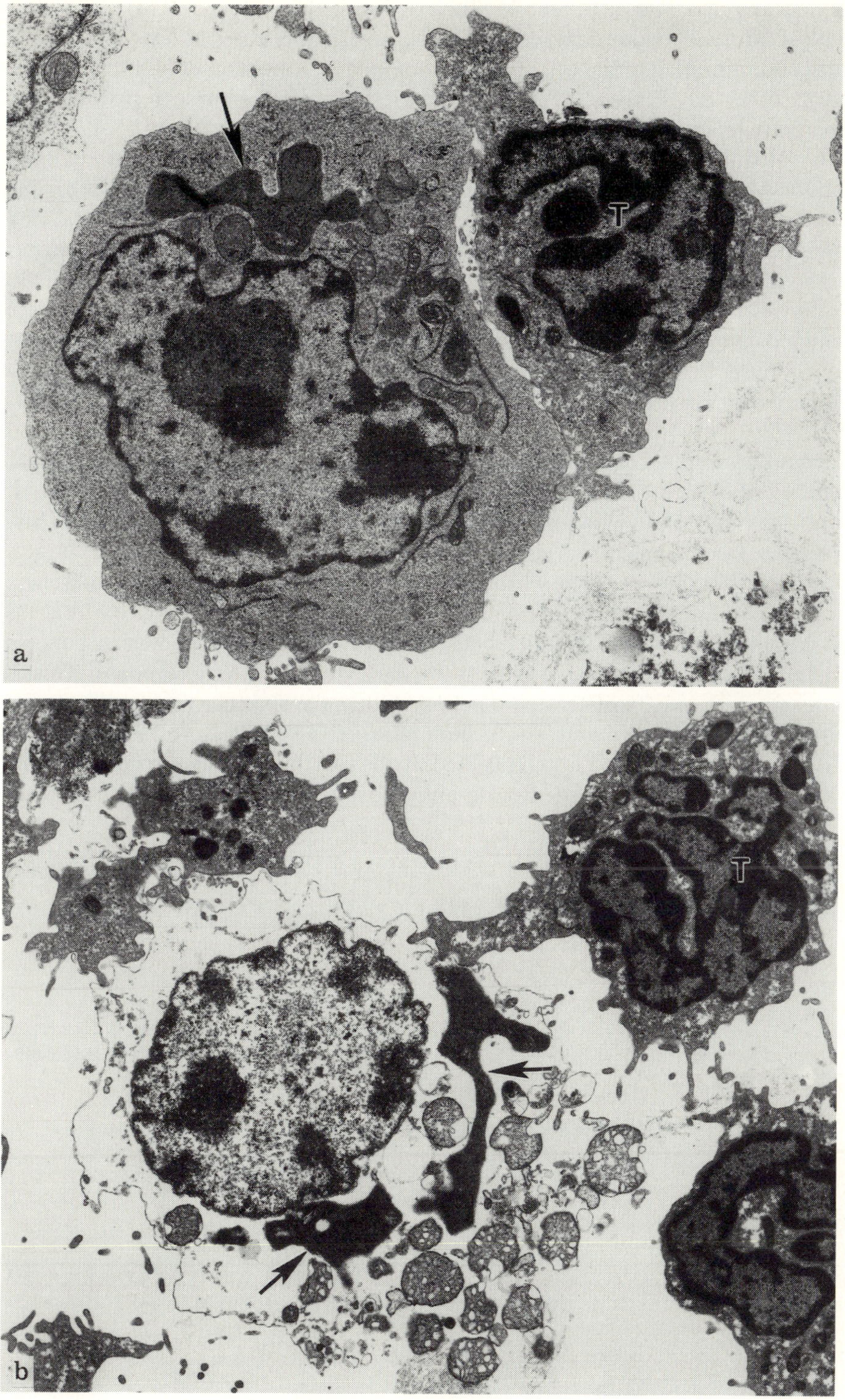
T
a
T
b

cell lines infected with either the Muguga or Marikebuni stocks (B.M. GODDEERIS and W.I. MORRISON, unpublished data), whereas in other cases at least some of the Marikebuni-infected target cell lines were not killed (GODDEERIS et al. 1986b). Thus, as was observed in vivo, the parasite strain specificity of the cytotoxic T cells apparently differed between individual cattle.

Cytotoxic T-cell clones have been derived from only one animal immunised with the Marikebuni stock. These clones killed target cells infected with either the Muguga or Marikebuni parasites (MORRISON et al. 1987a). The level of killing varied from one target cell to another, but this was shown to be due to cyclical changes in the target cells rather than heterogeneity within the individual cell lines. Clones restricted by class I molecules encoded by both MHC haplotypes were identified. Clones restricted by the same specificities (w6.2 and KN104) had also been derived from animals immunised with Muguga. Thus, it was possible to compare the parasite strain specificities of these clones using the same target cells. The results with two pairs of clones are shown in Table 2. The w6.2-restricted clones from animals immunised with Muguga or Marikebuni exhibited similar strain specificities in that they killed target cells infected with either parasite (B.M. GODDEERIS and W.I. MORRISON, unpublished data). By contrast, one KN104-restricted T-cell clone from the Marikebuni-immunised animal killed targets infected with either parasite whereas similarly restricted clones derived from a Muguga-immune animal were specific for targets infected with Muguga (GODDEERIS and MORRISON 1988b). The latter finding indicates that the immunising parasite can influence the antigenic specificity of the cytotoxic T-cell response. This is consistent with results of cross-protection in that the specificity of the immunity induced by the Muguga and Marikebuni parasites also differs.

However, the situation is complicated by the fact that, at least in the case of the Marikebuni stock, the parasite stock is antigenically and genetically heterogeneous.

Table 2. Influence of the immunising parasite stock on the parasite strain specificity of cytotoxic T-cell clones derived from immue cattle

Donor animal (MHC phenotype)	Immunising parasite stock	T-cell clone	Restricting MHC specificity[a]	Percent cytotoxicity on infected target cells of animal[b]			
				D409 (KN104/w7)		D247 (w6.2/w7)	
				Muguga	Marikebuni	Muguga	Marikebuni
C887 (KN104/w6.2)	Marikebuni	T21.7	KN104	32	35	0	2
		T19.7	w6.2	1	2	40	32
B641 (KN104/ KN18)	Muguga	T20.40	KN104	72	0	—	—
D232 (w2/w6.2)	Muguga	T23.110	w6.2	—	—	62	41

[a] The cytotoxicity of clones T21.7 and T20.40 was specifically inhibited by MAb IL-A4, which reacts with the KN104 specificity, and that of clones T19.7 and T23.110 was inhibited by MAb B4/18 which reacts with all w6$^+$ animals

[b] Results of cytotoxicity obtained at an effector to target ratio of 2:1 in a 4-h ^{51}Cr-release assay are presented

Thus, using MAbs specific for a *Theileria* antigen which differs in molecular weight between parasite populations, it has been possible to demonstrate four different forms of the antigen in cloned cell lines derived from the Marikebuni stock (B.M. GODDEERIS and P.G. TOYE, unpublished data). In some instances, cytotoxic T-cell clones generated from Muguga-immunised cattle could also distinguish between these cell lines infected with different Marikebuni parasites.

5.3 Influence of MHC Phenotype on Strain Specificity of the Cytotoxic T cells

There is considerable heterogeneity in the strain-specificity of the cytotoxic T-cell response and the immunity induced by the *T. parva* (Muguga) parasite. One factor which is likely to contribute to this is the MHC phenotype of the animal. In order to address this issue, we have analysed the strain specificity of cytotoxic T-cell clones which differed in MHC restriction specificity but originated from the same animal (B.M. GODDEERIS et al., submitted for publication). The restriction specificities were determined in the same way as for effector cells generated in vivo, i.e. by testing the effectors on panels of target cells of defined phenotypes and by inhibition with MAb specific for polymorphic class I determinants. Parasite strain specificity was evaluated on target cell lines infected with different Marikebuni parasites on the same animal cell background.

The first point to make is that sets of clones which exhibited similar MHC restriction specificities also had the same parasite strain specificity. By contrast, clones from the same animal restricted by different MHC determinants showed different strain specificities. The results with two representative clones from an animal immunised with *T. parva* (Muguga) are shown in Table 3. In each instance, the clones were assayed on one Muguga-infected target cell and on two different Marikebuni-infected target cells on the same animal cell background. These findings provide convincing evidence that the restricting MHC molecules, by selecting particular antigenic epitopes, can influence the parasite strain specificity of the T-cell response. Similar observations have been made in the cytotoxic T-cell responses of mice to influenza A viruses (VITIELLO and SHERMAN 1983). The influence of the MHC

Table 3. Influence of the restricting MHC molecule on parasite strain specificity of cytotoxic T-cell clones derived from an animal immunised with *T. parva* (Muguga)

Donor animal (MHC phenotype)	T-cell clone	Restricting MHC specificity	Percent cytotoxicity on autologous cells infected with:[a]		
			Muguga	Marikebuni 5	Marikebuni 16
C196 (w6/w7)	T26.20	w7	37	4	23
	T26.44	Undefined molecule on w6 haplotype	63	31	0

[a]Results of cytotoxicity obtained at an effector to target ratio of 2:1 in a 4-h ^{51}Cr-release assay are presented. Differences in the parasites within the Marikebuni 5 and Marikebuni 16 cell lines were detected with parasite-specific MAb

on selection of antigenic epitopes may be due either to differences within the T-cell repertoires in the frequencies of T cells specific for certain antigen-MHC combinations or to differences in the capacity of processed antigenic peptides to associate with different MHC class I molecules.

6 Concluding Remarks

Information on the kinetics and specificity of the cytotoxic T-cell response of cattle to *T. parva* indicates that the response is important in mediating immunity. Our studies have shown that the immunising parasite population and the MHC phenotype of the animal can have an influence on the parasite strain specificity of the cytotoxic T-cell response. The immunity engendered in cattle by infection and treatment with one stock of *T. parva* also displays a degree of strain specificity. However, since the parasite stocks currently under study are not antigenically homogeneous, definitive evidence for a correlation between specificity of the cytotoxic T-cell response and protection must await experiments with cloned populations of parasites.

Identification and characterisation of the antigens recognised by the cytotoxic T cells is essential in order to define the molecular basis of the antigenic differences between parasite populations and to explore the immunogenicity of such antigens. In view of the available evidence that the T cells are exquisitely specific for parasitised cells and exhibit parasite strain specificity, it seems likely that the target antigens are encoded by the parasite. The current thinking that antigens within the cytosol of cells tend to be processed and presented in the context of MHC class I molecules (Moore et al. 1988) is also consistent with the concept that the T cells recognise a parasite-derived antigen, since the *Theileria* parasite lies free within the cytoplasm of the host cell and therefore can presumably secrete or shed proteins directly into the cytosol.

The *Theileria* parasite is a relatively complex organism, having a genome of almost 10^7 base pairs (Morzaria et al. 1988). Over 200 proteins have been detected in two-dimensional gels prepared from lysates of radiolabelled purified schizonts (Sugimoto et al., in press). Strategies must, therefore, be devised for identification of, T-cell target antigens within this complex mixture. As already alluded to, antibodies are unlikely to detect antigens on the cell surface in a form in which they are recognised by T cells. Therefore, the parasite-specific T cells themselves must be used as screening reagents. In the case of class II restricted T cells, this can readily be done by examining the response of T cells to soluble antigenic fractions added to antigen-presenting cells. Indeed, $BoT4^+$ T-cell cultures specific for *T. parva*-infected cells, generated in vitro from immune cattle, have been shown to proliferate specifically in response to crude antigenic extracts from parasitised cells (Brown et al., in press). By contrast, class I restricted T cells generally recognise only antigens that are actively being synthesised within the presenting cells (L.A. Morrison et al. 1986) or are artificially introduced into the cytosol (Moore et al. 1988).

Consequently, the strategy to identify these target antigens is to isolate candidate parasite proteins or genes and determine whether the proteins or gene products are recognised by T cells following introduction, by appropriate means, into mammalian cells expressing the relevant bovine MHC molecules.

References

Baldwin CL, Goddeeris BM, Morrison WI (1987) Bovine helper T-cell clones specific for lymphocytes infected with *Theileria parva* (Muguga). Parasite Immunol 9: 499–513

Baldwin CL, Black SJ, Brown WC, Conrad PA, Goddeeris BM, Kinuthia SW, Lalor PA, MacHugh ND, Morrison WI, Morzaria SP, Naessens J, Newson J (1988) Bovine T cells, B cells, and null cells are transformed by the protozoan parasite *Theileria parva*. Infect Immun 56: 462–467

Brown CGD (1983) *Theileria*. In: Jenson JB (ed) In vitro culture of protozoan parasites. CRC, Boca Raton Fl, pp 243-284

Brown CGD, Stagg DA, Purnell RE, Kanhai GK, Payne RC (1973) Infection and transformation of bovine lymphoid cells in vitro by infective particles of *Theileria parva*. Nature 245: 101–103

Brown WC, Logan KS (1986) Bovine T-cell clones infected with *Theileria parva* produce a factor with IL 2-like activity. Parasite Immunol 8: 189–192

Brown WC, Sugimoto C, Grab DJ *Theileria parva*: bovine helper T cell clones specific for both infected lymphocytes and schizont membrane antigens. Exp Parasitol (in press)

Buller RML, Holmes KL, Hugin A, Frederickson TN, Morse HC (1987) Induction of cytotoxic T-cell responses in vivo in the absence of CD4 helper cells. Nature 328: 77–79

Conrad PA, Iams K, Brown WC, Sohanpal B, Ole-MoiYoi OK (1987) DNA probes detect genomic diversity in *Theileria parva* stocks. Mol Biochem Parasitol 25: 213–226

Conrad PA, Baldwin CL, Brown WC, Sohanpal B, Dolan TT, Goddeeris BM, DeMartini JC, ole-MoiYoi OK Infection of bovine T cell clones with genotypically distinct *Theileria parva* parasites and analysis of their cell surface phenotype. Parasitology (in press)

Creemers P (1982) Lack of reactivity of sera from *Theileria parva*-infected and recovered cattle against cell membrane antigens of *Theileria parva* transformed cell lines. Vet Immunol Immunopathol 3: 427–438

Dobbelaere DAE, Coquerelle TM, Roditi LJ, Eichhorn M, Williams RO (1988) *Theileria parva* infection induced autocrine growth of bovine lymphocytes. Proc Natl Acad Sci USA 85: 4730–4734

Emery DL (1981) Adoptive transfer of immunity to infection with *Theileria parva* (East Coast fever) between cattle twins. Res Vet Sci 30: 364–367

Emery DL, Eugui EM, Nelson RT, Tenywa T (1981) Cell-mediated immune responses to *Theileria parva* (East Coast fever) during immunization and lethal infections in cattle. Immunology 43: 323-335

Emery DL, MacHugh ND, Morrison WI (1988) *Theileria parva* (Muguga) infects bovine T lymphocytes in vivo and induces co-expression of BoT4 and BoT8. Parasite Immunol 10: 379–391

Eugui EM, Emery DL (1981) Genetically restricted cell-mediated cytotoxicity in cattle immune to *Theileria parva*. Nature 290: 251–254

Fawcett D, Musoke A, Voigt W (1984) Interaction of sporozoites of *Theileria parva* with bovine lymphocytes in vitro. 1. Early events after invasion. Tissue Cell 16: 873–884

Goddeeris BM, Morrison WI (1987) The bovine autologous *Theileria* mixed leucocyte reaction: influence of monocytes and phenotype of the parasitised stimulator cell on proliferation and parasite specificity. Immunology 60: 63–69

Goddeeris BM, Morrison WI (1988a) Techniques for the generation, cloning and characterization of bovine cytotoxic T cells specific for the protozoan *Theileria parva*. J Tissue Cult Methods 11: 101–110

Goddeeris BM, Morrison WI (1988b) *Theileria*-specific cytotoxic T cell clones: parasite stock specificity in relation to cross-protection. Ann NY Acad Sci 532: 459–461

Goddeeris BM, Morrison WI, Teale AJ (1986a) Generation of bovine cytotoxic cell lines specific for cells infected with the protozoan parasite *Theileria parva* and restricted by products of the major histocompatibility complex. Eur J Immunol 16: 1243–1249

Goddeeris BM, Morrison WI, Teale AJ, Bensaid A, Baldwin CL (1986b) Bovine cytotoxic T-cell clones specific for cells infected with the protozoan parasite *Theileria parva*: parasite strain specificity and class I major histocompatibility complex restriction. Proc Natl Acad Sci USA 83: 5238–5242

Heeg K, Steeg C, Hardt C, Wagner H (1987a) Identification of interleukin 2-producing T helper cells within murine Lyt-2^+ T lymphocytes: frequency, specificity and clonal segregation from Lyt-2^+ precursors of cytotoxic T lymphocytes. Eur J Immunol 17: 229–236

Heeg K, Steeg C, Schmitt J, Wagner H (1987b) Frequency analysis of class I MHC-reactive Lyt-2^+ and class II MHC-reactive L3T4^+ IL2-secreting T lymphocytes. J Immunol 138: 4121–4127

Hulliger L, Wilde JKH, Brown CGD, Turner L (1964) Mode of multiplication of *Theileria* in cultures of bovine lymphocytic cells. Nature 203: 728–730

Irvin AD (1985) Immunisation against theileriosis in Africa. International Laboratory for Research on Animal Diseases, Nairobi, pp 1–167

Irvin AD, Morrison WI (1987) Immunopathology, immunology and immunoprophylaxis of *Theileria* infections. In: Soulsby EJL (ed) Immune responses in parasitic infections: immunology, immunopathology and immunoprophylaxis, vol 3. CRC, Boca Raton Fl, pp 223–274

Irvin AD, Dobbelaere DAE, Mwamachi EM, Minami T, Spooner PR, Ocama JGR (1983) Immunisation against East Coast fever: correlation between monoclonal antibody profiles of *Theileria parva* stocks and cross immunity in vivo. Res Vet Sci 35: 341–346

Jenni LM Marti S, Schweizer J, Betschart B, Le Page RWF, Wells JM, Tait A, Paindavoine P, Pays E, Steinert M (1986) Hybrid formation between African trypanosomes during cyclical transmission. Nature 322: 173–175

Melhorn H, Schein E (1976) Electronenmikroskopische Untersuchungen an Entwicklungsstadien von *Theileria parva* im Darm der Überträgerzecke *Hyalomma anatolicum excavatum*. Tropenmed Parasitol 27: 182–191

Moore MW, Carbone FR, Bevan MJ (1988) Introduction of soluble protein into the class I pathway of antigen processing and presentation. Cell 54: 777–785

Morrison LA, Lukacher AE, Braciale VL, Fan DP, Braciale TJ (1986) Differences in antigen presentation to MHC class I- and class II-restricted influenza virus-specific cytolytic T lymphocyte clones. J Exp Med 163: 903–921

Morrison WI, Buscher G, Murray M, Emery DL, Masake RA, Cook RH, Wells PW (1981) *Theileria* parva: kinetics of infection in the lymphoid system of cattle. Exp Parasitol 52: 248–260

Morrison WI, Lalor PA, Goddeeris BM, Teale AJ (1986) Theileriosis: antigens and host-parasite interactions. In: Pearson TW (ed) Parasite antigens: toward new strategies for vaccines. Dekker, New York, pp 167–213

Morrison WI, Goddeeris BM, Teale AJ (1987a) Bovine cytotoxic T cell clones which recognize lymphoblasts infected with two antigenically different stocks of the protozoan parasite *Theileria parva*. Eur J Immunol 17: 1703–1709

Morrison WI, Goddeeris BM, Teale AJ, Groocock CM, Kemp SJ, Stagg DA (1987b) Cytotoxic T-cells elicited in cattle challenged with *Theileria parva* (Muguga): evidence for restriction by class I MHC determinants and parasite strain specificity. Parasite Immunol 9: 563–578

Morzaria SP, Young J, Bensaid A, Iams K, Musoke AJ, Sugimoto C (1988) Characterization of *T. parva* stocks using contour clamped homogeneous electric fields and field inversion gel electrophoresis. ILRAD Annu Sci Rep 1987: 8–9

Muhammed WI, Lauerman LH, Johnson LW (1975) Effect of humoral antibodies on the course of *Theileria parva* infection (East Coast fever) of cattle. Am J Vet Res 36: 399–402

Musoke AJ, Nantulya VM, Buscher G, Masake RA, Otim B (1982) Bovine immune response to *Theileria parva*: neutralizing antibodies to sporozoites. Immunology 45: 663–668

Neitz WO (1953) Aureomycin in *Theileria parva* infection. Nature 171: 34–35

Newson J, Naessens J, Stagg DA, Black SJ (1986) A cell surface antigen associated with *Theileria parva lawrencei*-infected bovine lymphoid cells. Parasite Immunol 8: 149–158

Pearson TW, Lundin LB, Dolan TT, Stagg DA (1979) Cell-mediated immunity to *Theileria*-transformed cell lines. Nature 281: 678–680

Pinder M, Kar S, Mayor-Withey KS, Lundin LB, Roelants GE (1981) Proliferation and lymphocyte stimulatory capacity of *Theileria*-infected lymphoblastoid cells before and after the elimination of intracellular parasites. Immunology 44: 51–60

Radley DE, Brown CGD, Burridge MJ, Cunningham MP, Kirimi IM, Purnell RE, Young AS (1975a) East Coast fever. 1. Chemoprophylactic immunization of cattle against *Theileria parva* (Muguga) and five theileria strains. Vet Parasitol 1: 35–41

Radley DE, Brown CGD, Cunningham MP, Kimber CD, Musisi FL, Payne RC, Purnell RE, Stagg SM, Young AS (1975b) East Coast fever. 3. Chemoprophylactic immunization of cattle using oxytetracycline and a combination of theileria strains. Vet Parasitol 1: 51–60

Radley DE, Brown CDG, Cunningham MP, Kimber CD, Musisi FL, Purnell RE, Stagg SM (1975c) East Coast fever: challenge of immunised cattle by prolonged exposure to infected ticks. Vet Rec 96: 525–528

Radley DE, Young AS, Brown CGD, Burridge MJ, Cunningham MP, Musisi FL, Purnell RE (1975d) East Coast fever. 2. Cross-immunity trials with a Kenya strain or *Theileria lawrencei*. Vet Parasitol 1: 43–50

Schein E, Warnecke M, Kirmse P (1977) The development of *Theileria parva* (Theiler 1904) in the gut of *Rhipicephalus appendiculatus*. Parasitology 75: 309–316

Shapiro SZ, Fujisaki K, Morzaria SP, Webster P, Fujinaga T, Spooner PR, Irvin AD (1987) A life cycle stage-specific antigen of *Theileria parva* recognised by anti-macroschizont monoclonal antibodies. Parasitology 94: 29–37

Sprent J, Schaefer M, Lo D, Korngold R (1986) Functions of purified L3T4$^+$ and Lyt-2$^+$ cells in vitro and in vivo. Immunol Rev 91: 195–218

Sugimoto C, Conrad PA, Mutharia L, Dolan TT, Brown WC, Goddeeris BM, Pearson TW Phenotypic characterization of *Theileria parva* schizonts by two-dimensional gel electrophoresis. Parasitol Res (in press)

Teale AJ, Kemp SJ, Young F, Spooner RL (1983) Selection of major histocompatibility type (BoLA) of lymphoid cells derived from a bovine chimaera and transformed by *Theileria* parasites. Parasite Immunol 5: 329–336

Townsend ARM, Rothbard J, Botch FM, Bahadur G, Wraith D, McMichael AJ (1986) The epitopes of influenza nucleoprotein recognized by cytotoxic T lymphocytes can be defined with short synthetic peptides. Cell 44: 959–968

Vitiello A, Sherman LA (1983) Recognition of influenza-infected cells by cytolytic T lymphocyte clones: determinant selection by class I restriction elements. J Immunol 131: 1635–1640

Walliker D, Quakyi IA, Wellems TE, McCutchan TF, Szarfman A, London WT, Corcoran LM, Burkot TR, Carter R (1987) Genetic analysis of the human malaria parasite *Plasmodium falciparum*. Science 236: 1661–1666

Bacteria

T-Lymphocytes in Leprosy Lesions*

V. MEHRA[1] and R.L. MODLIN[2]

1 Introduction

Leprosy, a chronic infectious disease caused by *Mycobacterium leprae*, has provided extraordinary possibilities for gaining insight into immunoregulatory mechanisms in man (BLOOM 1986). The disease is not a single entity but rather presents a spectrum of clinical and histopathological manifestations that correlate extraordinarily well with cell-mediated immunity (RIDLEY and JOPLING 1966). Patients at the tuberculoid end of the spectrum characteristically have few localized lesions, containing rare organisms, and mount a strong cell-mediated immune response that ultimately kills and clears the bacilli. At the other end of the spectrum, patients with the lepromatous form have numerous disseminated skin lesions containing enormously high numbers of acid-fast bacilli and show specific immunological unresponsiveness to antigens of *M. leprae,* in vivo and in vitro (BLOOM and MEHRA 1984). Antibodies to *M. leprae* are found throughout the spectrum, the highest levels occurring in the lepromatous disease, indicating that they are unlikely to play a major role in protection. On the other hand, there is a striking inverse correlation between level of cell-mediated immunity to antigens of *M. leprae* and the growth of the organism in the tissues. The selective and specific cell-mediated unresponsiveness at the lepromatous end of the spectrum to antigens of *M. leprae*, provides a unique opportunity for exploring mechanisms of tolerance in man (BLOOM and MEHRA 1984).

Although most of the immunological studies have been conducted with peripheral blood lymphocytes, the focal point of the immune response to *M. leprae* is the tissue granuloma, a collection of lymphocytes and macrophages. To address questions concerning the antigen specificity and immunological functions in lesions of human infectious disease, the mechanism by which T-suppressor cells may contribute to immunological unresponsiveness and the identification of a T-cell phenotype that may be crucial to protection, we designed studies to delineate various T-lymphocytes infiltrating leprosy lesions in situ and their function in vitro.

* Supported by grants from the National Institutes of Health (AI22553, AI07118, AI02111, AI23545), the UNDP/World Bank/World Health Organization Special Programme for Research and Training in Tropical Diseases (IMMLEP and THELEP), National Hansen's Disease Center, Knights of St. Lazarus of Jerusalem, and the Drown Foundation

[1] Department of Microbiology and Immunology, Albert Einstein College of Medicine, Bronx, NY, USA

[2] Section of Dermatology and Department of Pathology, University of Southern California School of Medicine, Los Angeles, CA, USA

Current Topics in Microbiology and Immunology, Vol. 155

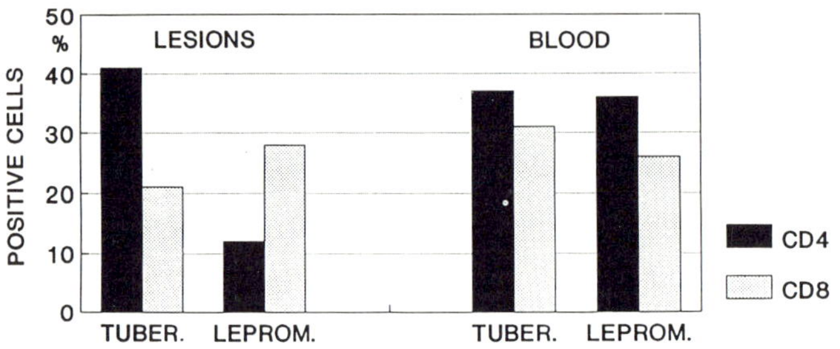

Fig. 1. T-lymphocyte subsets in the lesions and blood of leprosy patients

2 Identification of T-Lymphocytes in Lesions

The advent of monoclonal antibodies directed against T-lymphocyte subpopulations has permitted the characterization of cells in leprosy lesions of skin and nerves. Several investigators have used these antibodies to visualize the T-lymphocytes in situ, in frozen sections of biopsy specimens, by immunoperoxidase or immunofluorescence techniques (Modlin et al. 1982, 1983a, b, c, 1984, 1985, 1986c; van Voorhis et al. 1982; Narayanan et al. 1983, 1984; Kato et al. 1983; Wallach et al. 1984; Sarno et al. 1984; Longley et al. 1985; Nilsen et al. 1986). These studies indicate striking differences in the CD4:CD8 (T-helper/inducer:T-suppressor/cytotoxic) ratio at the poles of the leprosy spectrum. The data from all studies indicate that in tuberculoid leprosy lesions the CD4 population predominates with a CD4:CD8 ratio of 1.9:1, and in lepromatous lesions the CD8 population predominates with a CD4:CD8 ratio of 0.6:1. It is intriguing that the CD4:CD8 ratios in the lesions are independent of those in the blood of the patients (Modlin et al. 1986a; Fig. 1). This suggests that there is some selective migration of cells into, proliferation within, or retention in lesions. Furthermore, it underscores the importance of studying these cells at sites of disease activity rather than the peripheral blood.

3 Subpopulations of T-Lymphocyte Subsets

Recently, the CD4 and CD8 subsets have been further divided into subpopulations by new monoclonal antibodies (Beverley 1986; Sanders et al. 1988; Yamada et al. 1985). $CD8^+$ cells that bear the CD28 marker have cytotoxic function, and those that are $CD28^-$ have suppressor function in vitro. Similarly, evidence suggests that $CD4^+$ cells bearing the CDw29 or CD45 markers belong to a T-helper/memory subpopulation whereas those expressing CD45R or Leu8 antigens comprise a population of naive (or suppressor-inducer) T cells. Using these monoclonal

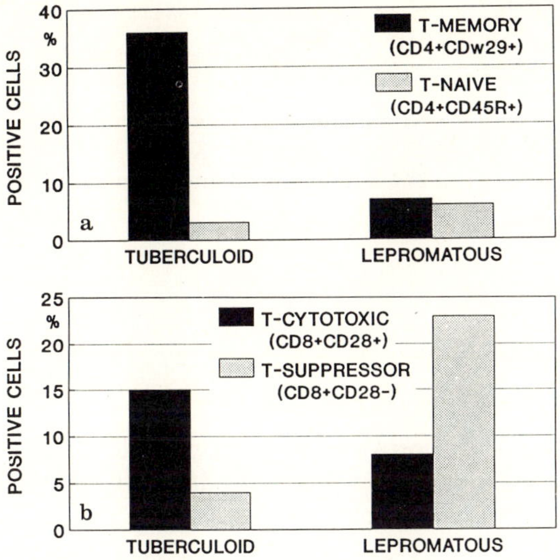

Fig. 2a, b. Subpopulations of CD4 and CD8 subsets in leprosy lesions

antibodies to distinguish CD4 and CD8 subpopulations in granulomas, striking differences in the proportions and distribution of these subsets were observed (MODLIN et al. 1988; Fig. 2).

While the CD4:CD8 ratio is 2:1 both in the blood and lesions of tuberculoid patients, the tissue population does not represent random filtrate from blood. The T-helper/memory:T-naive ratio was 1:1 in blood but 14:1 in the lesions. In contrast, in the lepromatous lesions one-half of the $CD4^+$ cells belong to the T-naive subset, with the majority of $CD8^+$ cells belonging to the T-suppressor subset. $CD8^+$ cells of the T-cytotoxic phenotype are predominant in tuberculoid lesions.

4 Immunologic Microenvironments

Although the relative percentages of T-lymphocytes and their subsets in leprosy lesions is of great interest, their localization in the tuberculoid granuloma into distinct microenvironments is even more intriguing. We reported (MODLIN et al. 1982, 1983c) the microanatomic association of $CD4^+$ cells with macrophages in the core of the granuloma with the relative restriction of $CD8^+$ cells to the mantle surrounding the granuloma, which was also confirmed by others (NARAYANAN et al. 1983; WALLACH et al. 1984; LONGLEY et al. 1985). In lepromatous granulomas the $CD8^+$ cells were admixed with macrophages and $CD4^+$ cells which could facilitate suppression of the cell-mediated immune response.

Double immunostaining of CD4 subpopulations revealed that the tuberculoid granuloma was divided into distinct immunological microenvironments (MODLIN et al. 1988). The $CD4^+$ cells present in the center of the granuloma were of the T-helper/memory phenotype. Since they are located near macrophages, it is conceivable that they may play a role in mediating macrophage localization, activation, and maturation that leads to restriction or elimination of the pathogen. The T-naive or suppressor-inducer subset was localized to the mantle surrounding the granuloma, near $CD8^+$ cells, where they perhaps restrict the cell-mediated immune response from causing extensive tissue damage.

5 Functional Activity of T-Lymphocytes

Although phenotyping of lymphocytes in leprosy lesions has provided useful information about the nature of cells present in the granulomas, delineation of the immune function of these cells is of potentially greater interest.

5.1 Detection of Functional Populations in Lesions by In Situ Hybridization to Detect Specific mRNA

The immunoperoxidase technique has been used successfully by ourselves (Modlin et al. 1984) and Longley et al. (1985) to detect interleukin 2 (IL-2), a lymphokine necessary for T-cell proliferation in leprosy lesions. The number of IL-2 containing cells was an order of magnitude greater in tuberculoid lesions than in lepromatous lesions (Fig. 3). However, the immunoperoxidase technique has been relatively unsuccessful in determining the presence of other lymphokines in lesions. The technique of in situ hybridization allows for the detection of mRNA coding for proteins that are characteristic of a particular functional population. Since interferon-γ (IFN-γ) has been shown to facilitate the intracellular killing of mycobacteria in vitro and in vivo (Rook et al. 1986; Nathan et al. 1986), we examined leprosy skin biopsy specimens for the presence of mRNA encoding for IFN-γ (Cooper et al. 1989). Cells showing hybridization were more numerous in tuberculoid lesions in comparison to lepromatous lesions. The percentages of positive cells similar to that seen using the anti-IL-2 monoclonal antibody.

Further, we studied lesions for the presence of T cells of potential cytotoxic function using a riboprobe for an enzymatic marker associated with cytotoxic cells, serine esterase (huHF). Cells positive for huHF were more numerous in tuberculoid lesions as compared to lepromatous lesions. T-cytotoxic cells are thought to contribute to host defenses against mycobacterial infection by lysing infected targets in vitro (Mustafa and Godal 1987). In lesions, IFN-γ production may enhance the cytolytic action of $CD4^+$ class II restricted killer cells by inducing major histocompatibility complex (MHC) expression on targets (Kaufmann et al. 1987). The lysis of these infected targets in tuberculoid lesions may then eventuate in the elimination of bacilli, allowing the dilution of organisms from heavily parasitized macrophages into fresh IFN-γ activated phagocytes, where destruction can then

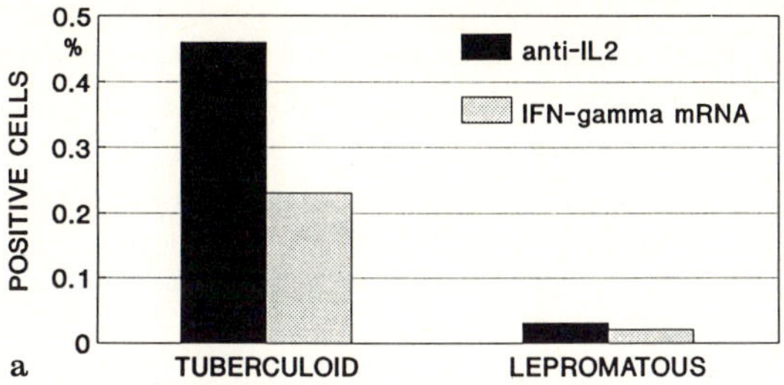

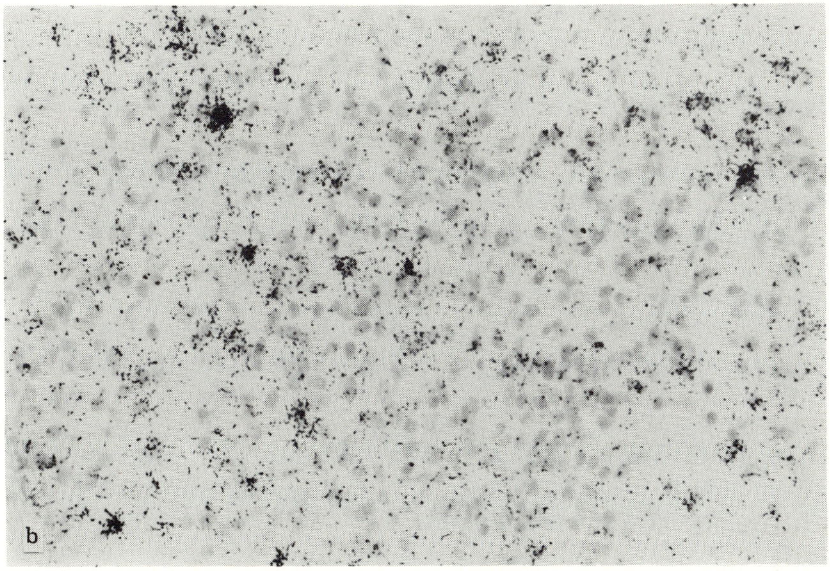

Fig. 3a, b. Lymphokines in leprosy lesions. **a** Percentage of positive cells in leprosy lesions identified with an anti-IL-2 monoclonal antibody and those identified as containing mRNA coding for IFN-γ. **b** Photomicrograph of a leprosy lesions showing IFN-γ mRNA containing cells as detected by in situ hybridization using an 35S-labelled probe

take place. In lepromatous lesions, serine esterase positive cells were observed, albeit fewer than in tuberculoid lesions. This raises the question of how cells bearing genotypic markers of cytotoxicity can be present yet bacillary proliferation proceed unchecked. One cannot rule out the possibility that some effector molecule other than serine esterase is required for cytotoxicity (Ferguson et al. 1988). If the cells in lepromatous lesions are capable of cytolysis, the levels of IFN-γ produced locally may be insufficient to activate fresh macrophages to kill bacilli.

5.2 Function of Blood and Tissue-Derived T-Helper Cells

Methods were developed for isolating lymphocytes from the leprosy lesions in order to measure their function in vitro (Modlin et al. 1986a, b, d,1988). Limiting dilution analysis of these tissue-extracted T-lymphocytes was undertaken in order to determine the precursor frequency of antigen-reactive T-lymphocytes (Modlin et al. 1988). Of T-lymphocytes from tuberculoid leprosy lesions, 2% were capable of proliferation in response to *M. leprae* while only 0.02% of peripheral blood lymphocytes were reactive to the same antigen preparation (Modlin et al. 1988). Thus, not only is there a 10-fold enrichment of T-helper/memory subset in tuberculoid lesions, but as much as a 100-fold enrichment in antigen reactive T-lymphocytes in the lesions.

We initially observed that T cells derived from peripheral blood of tuberculoid leprosy patients and lepromin skin test positive contacts proliferate in response to purified *M. leprae* cell walls (Melancon-Kaplan et al. 1988). Therefore, we wished to ascertain whether T cells in leprosy lesions have been activated by cell wall antigens in vivo during the natural course of their infection (Mehra et al. 1989). Accordingly, the T cells derived from tuberculoid lesions were expanded in the presence of IL-2 alone to select for cell activated in situ by antigenic stimulation and express IL-2 receptors. $CD4^+$ lines derived from tuberculoid leprosy lesions responded equally to whole *M. leprae* and cell walls but failed to respond to tetanus toxoid, confirming the specificity of the cells from the lesion (Fig. 4). $CD4^+$ lines similarly established from lepromatous lesions were unresponsive to all *M. leprae* antigen preparations.

Our earlier studies indicated that highly purified cell walls of *M. leprae*, essentially devoid of detectable amounts of lipids, carbohydrates, and soluble proteins, stimulated proliferation of T cells from tuberculoid patients/contacts as well as whole *M. leprae* and elicited delayed-type hypersensitivity in guinea-pigs and patients sensitized to *M. leprae* (Melancon-Kaplan et al. 1988; Hunter et al. 1989). This immunological activity was destroyed by pronase treatment, indicating that protein is a major contributor to cell-mediated immune reactivity to this pathogen.

In order to identify and characterize the individual cell wall antigens recognized by T cells of *M. leprae* responsive individuals, we employed *M. leprae*/cell wall reactive $CD4^+$ clones/lines (Hunter et al. 1989; Mehra et al. 1989). A major methodological advance in facilitating the identification of antigens recognized at

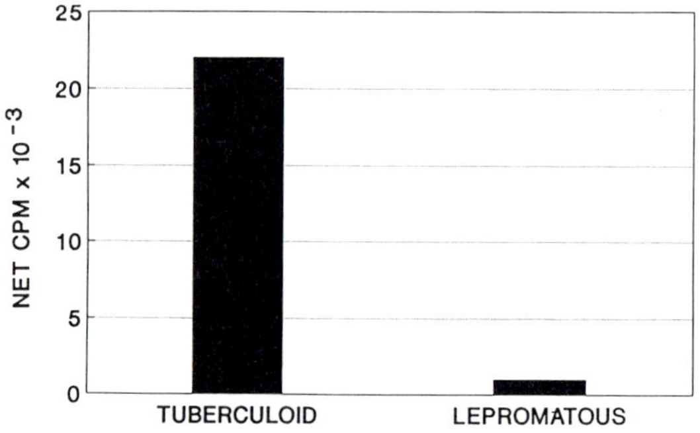

Fig. 4. Reactivity of $CD4^+$ T-cell lines from leprosy lesions to *M. leprae* cell wall. $CD4^+$ cells were extracted from lesions and cultured in the presence of IL-2 alone to expand those cells which had been stimulated in vivo to express IL-2 receptors

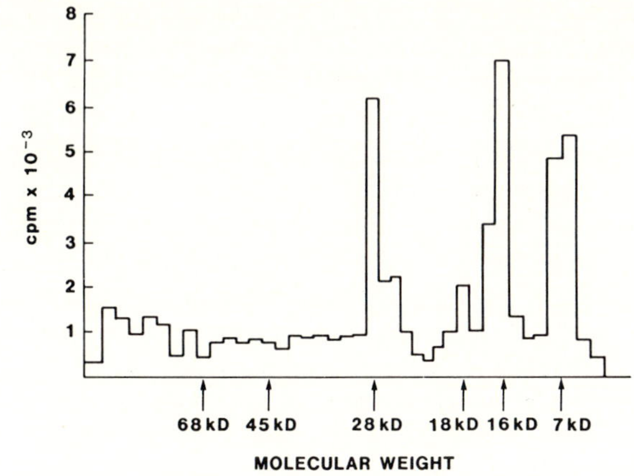

Fig. 5. T-cell Western blot of *M. leprae* cell wall reactive T-cell line. This line recognizes *M. leprae* proteins of molecular weight 7 kDa, 16 kDa, and 28 kDa

the T-cell level has been the development of the T-cell Western blot technique by Young and Lamb (YOUNG and LAMB 1986; LAMB and YOUNG 1987) and Abou-Zeid et al. (1987). The method involves separation of proteins from *M. leprae* sonicate by standard sodium dodecyl sulfate polyacrylamide gel electrophoresis (SDS-PAGE) and transfer onto nitrocellulose filter. The discrete molecular weight fractions can be tested for their ability to stimulate T-cell lines and clones after converting nitrocellulose membranes into fine antigen-bearing particles. On the assumption that sonic extracts of *M. leprae* contain cell wall protein antigens, T-cell lines previously established to cell walls were tested for their reactivity against *M. leprae* antigens separated on 5%–20% gradient SDS-PAGE gels. In 18 individuals tested, greatest reactivity was observed to proteins of molecular weight of 7 and 16 kDa (Fig. 5). The results indicate that the antigens or fragments of molecular weight 7, 16, 18, 28, and 65 kDa are components of the most highly purified cell wall protein preparations.

Since antigens of molecular weight 16 and 7 kDa from *M. leprae* have not been reported previously, we considered the possibility that they might be proteolytic fragments or subunits of larger proteins. T-cell clones reactive to 16- and 7-kDa polypeptides did not react with bands of any other size proteins present on the nitrocellulose blot, indicating that these two polypeptides of approximate M_r of 7 and 16 kDa are individual proteins and not fragments of larger proteins.

5.3 T-Suppressor Cells in the Blood and Lesions of Leprosy Patients

The most puzzling and fundamental immunological issue in lepromatous leprosy that remains unresolved is that of selective and specific unresponsiveness. As discussed earlier, most patients with lepromatous leprosy exhibit normal cell-mediated immunity to a variety of mycobacterial antigens, including purified protein derivative (PPD), while remaining totally unresponsive to antigens of

M. leprae. Since all known protein or glycoprotein antigens of *M. leprae* appear to be cross-reactive with antigens of other mycobacteria, how is it possible to respond to the cross-reactive antigens when they are associated with *M. tuberculosis* or bacillus Calmette-Guérin (BCG) and yet be totally unresponsive when these antigens are associated with *M. leprae*? We suggested the hypothesis that there might be one or a small number of unique epitopes associated with *M. leprae* capable of inducing suppression of the potentially cross-reactive helper cells (Mehra et al. 1979, 1980, 1982; Nelson et al. 1987). In order to test this, we examined the ability of *M. leprae* antigens to induce suppressor activity. Lacking HLA-matched individuals, the initial studies were conducted using *M. leprae* antigens (lepromin) to induce suppression of lymphocyte concanavalin A (Con A) responses at 72 h. In over 200 patients studied, suppression was found in 84% of lepromatous and borderline patients, but not in tuberculoid patients, contacts, or normal donors. Both adherent and nonadherent cell populations in the peripheral blood of lepromatous and borderline patients were capable of suppressing Con A responses. While macrophage-induced suppression is related to the extent of disease and is not antigen specific, the suppression induced by T cells was lepromin specific and was mediated by $CD8^+$ subsets of T cells. Of these $CD8^+$ cells, 50% expressed activation markers, namely Fc receptors and Ia antigens. Using the phenolic glycolipid unique to *M. leprae*, we observed that the glycolipid induced suppression of Con A responses to the same extent as whole *M. leprae* in lepromatous leprosy patients (Mehra et al. 1984).

Since lesions of lepromatous leprosy contain a high proportion of $CD8^+$ cells, it was critical to determine whether the cells infiltrating the lesions could manifest antigen-induced suppressor activity. We extracted $CD8^+$ cells from lesions to establish lines and clones, which were tested for their ability to induce suppression (Modlin et al. 1986a, d). Lines derived from lepromatous but not tuberculoid lesions were able to suppress mitogen responses of peripheral blood lymphocytes of normal donors only in the presence of *M. leprae* (Fig. 6; Modlin et al. 1986a). When $CD8^+$ clones derived from lepromatous lesions were tested for

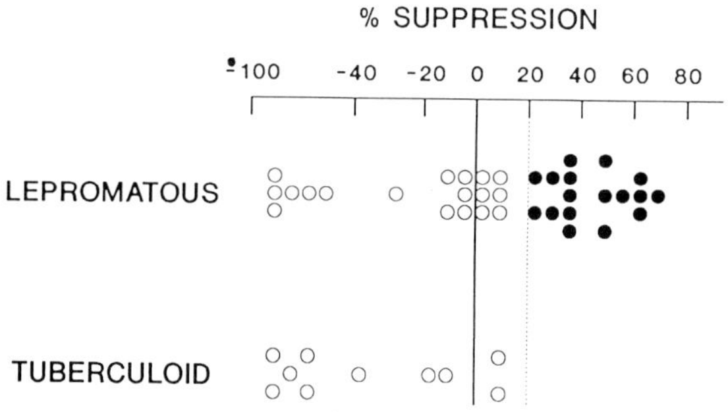

Fig. 6. *M. leprae* induced suppressor activity of $CD8^+$ T-cell lines derived from leprosy lesions. One-third of the $CD8^+$ lines from lepromatous lesions, but not tuberculoid lesions, could be induced to suppress by *M. leprae*

their ability to suppress the response of *M. leprae* specific $CD4^+$ clones from tuberculoid patients to lepromin, the suppressor activity was found to be restricted by MHC class II antigens (MODLIN et al. 1986d). The abundance of $CD8^+$ cells in lepromatous lesions, which appear to have T-suppressor activity in vitro, and close proximity to $CD4^+$ cells and macrophages, could result in unresponsiveness in vivo. While some previous efforts to detect antigen-specific suppression by lymphocytes from lepromatous patients have not been successful, it is gratifying to note that recently DE VRIES and his coworkers (OTTENHOFF et al. 1986) as well as SASAZUKI (personal communication) have not only demonstrated the suppression of lepromin responses by CD8 cells from lepromatous patients but have also observed it to be MHC class II restricted.

Further, the CD8 suppressor clones were examined for the presence and rearrangement of the antigen receptor (MODLIN et al. 1987). These T-suppressor clones were noted to rearrange T-cell receptor (TCR) β-genes, express messenger RNA for α- and β-chains, and express α, β heterodimer T-cell receptors on their cell surface. Immunohistological studies further demonstrated that the majority of $CD8^+$ cells in lepromatous lesions expressed the β-chain of the TCR in situ (MODLIN et al. 1987).

The very existence, nature, and function of T-suppressor cells remains a controversial subject in cellular immunology. In no system are the mechanisms known by which suppressor cells act to block specific antigen responses. However, the involvement of T-suppressor cells in the selective immunological unresponsiveness in leprosy has been critically tested at several levels.

1. The prevalence of T-suppressor cells in lepromatous but not tuberculoid patients indicates a stage-of-disease association correlated with their clinical condition (MEHRA et al. 1979)
2. $CD8^+$ T-cell lines and clones established directly from lepromatous lesions are found to suppress antigen and mitogen responses in vitro in an MHC class II restricted manner.
3. Appropriate chemotherapeutic treatment of lepromatous patients is associated with a concomitant decrease in T-suppressor activity.
4. Immunotherapeutic vaccination of lepromatous patients by Convit and his coworkers in Venezuela, with a mixture of killed *M. leprae* + BCG resulted in reduction of T-suppressor activity concomitant with clinical improvement (BLOOM and MEHRA 1984).
5. Depletion of $CD8^+$ cells from the peripheral blood of borderline lepromatous patients can restore *M. leprae* responsiveness in vitro (BLOOM and MEHRA 1984).
6. Antigen-specific T-suppressor lines and clones have been established from lepromatous lesions but not tuberculoid lesions (MODLIN et al. 1986a, d).
7. The mechanism of suppression in leprosy may be due to the ability of T-suppressor cells to negate or block induction of a second signal required for T-cell activation leading to a state of unresponsiveness (SALGAME et al. 1989).

These results support the view that the spectrum of leprosy represents a subtle regulatory balance of T-helper and T-suppressor cells within lesions that determines the ultimate course of the disease.

6 Reactional States

The immunological spectrum of leprosy is not static, as patients can undergo one of several reactions called "reactional states." Study of these dynamic reactions provide insight into the immunoregulatory mechanisms in leprosy, an added dimension to studies of the baseline spectrum.

Reversal reactions in leprosy are characterized by a reduction, or occasionally the elimination, of organisms from lesions with upgrading of the clinical classification associated with a sudden gain in cell-mediated immunity against *M. leprae*. Cells infiltrating the reversal reaction lesions contain mRNA coding for IFN-γ as well as human serine esterase and express cell surface antigenic determinants of the T-helper and T-cytotoxic subpopulations (Cooper et al. 1989). These results provide evidence that reversal reactions represent a naturally occurring delayed-type hypersensitivity reaction in leprosy.

Erythema nodosum leprosum (ENL) occurs in half the patients with lepromatous leprosy and is characterized histologically by neutrophilic and increased lymphocytic infiltration of bacilli-laden lepromatous granulomas. The relative increase in $CD4^+$ cells in the lesions of ENL patients compared to lepromatous leprosy patients suggests a cell-mediated immune mechanism (Modlin et al. 1983c). Furthermore, serial studies of lepromatous patients that developed ENL demonstrated a dynamic reversal of the helper:suppressor ratio during the reaction, with the predominance of T-helper/inducer cell phenotype (Modlin et al. 1986c). Analysis of ENL lesions revealed that the immune processes underlying its pathogenesis could clearly be differentiated from that of reversal reaction. Although phenotypic T-helper cells predominated in ENL lesions, the high levels of IFN-γ gene expression characteristic of reversal reactions were not observed (Cooper et al. 1989). ENL granulomas lacked the characteristic microanatomic separation of T-cell subpopulations found in tuberculoid and reversal reaction granulomas. In addition, the percentage of T-cytotoxic cells as measured by immunoperoxidase or in situ hybridization were relatively low in these ENL specimens.

It is tempting to speculate that the differences observed between reversal reactions and ENL reactions in leprosy can be envisioned as representing different dynamic events occurring in the lesions of the patients. Reversal reactions would appear to reflect a selective *increase* in $CD4^+$ IFN-γ producing and $CD4^+$ and/or $CD8^+$ cytotoxic T-lymphocyte activity in the lesions, with the number of $CD8^+$ T-suppressor cells remaining almost constant. In contrast, ENL reactions may be visualized as a transient *diminution* in T-suppressor activity, leading to partial augmentation of T-helper activity. We have reported a transient diminution of T-suppressor activity in vitro during ENL episodes (Modlin et al. 1986c). The diminution of T-suppressor regulation could account for the augmentation of both cell-mediated immunity and antibody formation characteristic of ENL reactions. However, ENL reactions would appear to lack significant numbers of lymphokine-producing cells and fail to exhibit a significant increase in cytotoxic T-lymphocytes. This picture could lead to the immune-complex disease symptoms associated with the syndrome, but without the massive killing of bacteria associated with reversal reactions.

7 TCR $\gamma\delta$ Cells in Leprosy Lesions

The majority of T cells bear the TCR $\alpha\beta$-complex which recognizes foreign antigen peptides only in the context of self MHC molecules. Such T cells function in a variety of effector roles and secrete cytokines that mediate the activation and differentiation of other cells in the immune system. Recently, a small subpopulation of T cells was found to bear a distinct TCR composed of γ and δ subunits (BRENNER et al. 1986). In contrast to the normal low frequency ($< 10\%$) of $\gamma\delta$-bearing cells in peripheral blood of leprosy patients, the frequency was increased by five- to eightfold in particular granulomatous reactions of leprosy, specifically reversal reactions and the Mitsuda reaction (the 3-week skin test to *M. leprae*) (MODLIN et al. 1989). TCR $\gamma\delta^+$-lymphocyte lines from these leprosy skin lesions were found to proliferate in vitro specifically to mycobacterial antigens. This reactivity to foreign antigens appears to require presentation in the context of self-molecules. Moreover, culture supernatants from activated $\gamma\delta$-T-lymphocytes induced adhesion and aggregation of bone marrow monocytes in the presence of GM-CSF, suggesting that products of $\gamma\delta$-bearing T cells may play a role in granuloma formation.

8 Conclusion

The study of T-cell subsets and their function in leprosy lesions continues to offer new insights into regulation of cell-mediated immunity in man. In addition, such studies provide a unique insight into the dynamics of the disease, leprosy. As we continue to learn from lesions, so we will continue to learn about leprosy and the immune response to pathogens in man.

Acknowledgements. We are deeply grateful to our research collaborators that contributed to many of the studies detailed in this manuscript. We give special thanks to Barry R. Bloom, Patrick J. Brennan, and Thomas H. Rea for their guidance and encouragement.

References

Abou-Zeid C, Filley E, Steele J, Rook GAW (1987) A simple new method for using antigens separated by polyacrylamide gel electrophoresis to stimulate lymphocytes in vitro after converting bands cut from western blots into antigen-bearing particles. J Immunol Methods 98: 5–10

Beverley PCL (1986) Human T cells subsets. Immunol Lett 14: 263–267

Bloom BR (1986) Learning from leprosy: a perspective on immunology and the third world. J Immunol 137: i–x

Bloom BR, Mehra V (1984) Immunological unresponsiveness in leprosy. Immunol Rev 80: 5–28

Brenner MB, McLean J, Dialynas DP, Strominger JL, Smith JA, Owen FL, Seidman JG, Ip S, Rosen F, Krangel MS (1986) Identification of a putative second T-cell receptor. Nature 322: 145–149

Cooper CL, Muller C, Sinchaisri T-A, Pirmez C, Chan J, Kaplan G, Young SMM, Weissman IL, Bloom BR, Rea TH, Modlin RL (1989) Analysis of naturally occurring delayed-type hypersensitivity reactions in leprosy by in situ hybridization. J Exp Med 169: 1565–1581
Ferguson WS, Verret CR, Reilly EB, Iannini MJ, Eisen HN (1988) Serine esterase and hemolytic activity in human cloned cytotoxic T lymphocytes. J Exp Med 167: 528–540
Hunter SW, McNeil M, Modlin RL, Mehra V, Bloom BR, Brennan PJ (1989) Isolation and characterization of the highly immunogenic cell wall-associated proteins of *Mycobacterium leprae*. J Immunol 142: 2873–2878
Kato H, Sanada K, Koseki M, Ozawa T (1983) Identification of lymphocyte subpopulations in cutaneous lesions of leprosy. Nippon Rai Gakkai Zasshi 52: 126–132
Kaufmann SHE, Hug E, Vath U, DeLibero G (1987) Specific lysis of *Listeria* monocytogenes-infected macrophages by class II-restricted L3T4$^+$ T cells. Eur J Immunol 17: 237–246
Lamb JR, Young DB (1987) A novel approach to the identification of T-cell epitopes in *Mycobacterium tuberculosis* using human T-lymphocyte clones. Immunology 60: 1–5
Longley J, Haregewoin A, Yemaneberhan T, van Diepen TW, Nsijbami J, Knowles D, Smith KA, Godal T (1985) In vivo responses to *Mycobacterium leprae:* antigen presentation, interleukin-2 production, and immune cell phenotypes in naturally occurring leprosy lesions. Int J Leprosy 53: 385–394
Mehra V, Mason LH, Fields JP, Bloom BR (1979) Lepromin-induced suppressor cells in patients with leprosy. J Immunol 123: 1813–1817
Mehra V, Mason LH, Rothman W, Reinherz E, Schlossman SF, Bloom BR (1980) Delineation of a human T cell subset responsible for lepromin-induced suppression in leprosy patients. J Immunol 125: 1183–1188
Mehra V, Convit J, Rubinstein A, Bloom BR (1982) Activated suppressor T cells in leprosy. J Immunol 129: 1946–1951
Mehra V, Brennan PJ, Rada E, Convit J, Bloom BR (1984) Lymphocyte suppression in leprosy induced by unique *M. leprae* glycolipid. Nature 308: 194–196
Mehra V, Bloom BR, Torigian VK, Mandich D, Reichel M, Young SMM, Salgame P, Convit J, Hunter SW, McNeil M, Brennan PJ, Rea TH, Modlin RL (1989) Characterization of *Mycobacterium leprae* cell wall-associated proteins using T-lymphocyte clones. J Immunol :
Melancon-Kaplan J, Hunter SW, McNeil M, Stewart C, Modlin RL, Rea TH, Convit J, Salgame P, Mehra V, Bloom BR, Brennan PJ (1988) Immunological significance of *Mycobacterium leprae* cell walls. Proc Natl Acad Sci USA 85: 1917–1921
Modlin RL, Hofman FM, Taylor CR, Rea TH (1982) In situ characterization of T lymphocyte subsets in leprosy granulomas [letter]. Int J Leprosy 50: 361–362
Modlin RL, Hofman FM, Meyer PR, Sharma OP, Taylor CR, Rea TH (1983a) In situ demonstration of T lymphocyte subsets in granulomatous inflammation: leprosy, rhinoscleroma and sarcoidosis. Clin Exp Immunol 51: 430–438
Modlin RL, Gebhard JF, Taylor CR, Rea TH (1983b) In situ characterization of T lymphocyte subsets in the reactional states of leprosy. Clin Exp Immunol 53: 17–24
Modlin RL, Hofman FM, Taylor CR, Rea TH (1983c) T lymphocyte subsets in the skin lesions of patients with leprosy. J Am Acad Dermatol 8: 182–189
Modlin RL, Hofman FM, Horwitz DA, Husmann LA, Gillis S, Taylor CR, Rea TH (1984) In situ identification of cells in human leprosy granulomas with monoclonal antibodies to interleukin 2 and its receptor. J Immunol 132: 3085–3090
Modlin RL, Bakke AC, Vaccaro SA, Horwitz DA, Taylor CR, Rea TH (1985) Tissue and blood T-lymphocyte subpopulations in erythema nodosum leprosum. Arch Dermatol 121: 216–219
Modlin RL, Mehra V, Wong L, Fujimiya Y, Chang W-C, Horwitz DA, Bloom BR, Rea TH, Pattengale PK (1986a) Suppressor T lymphocytes from lepromatous leprosy skin lesions. J Immunol 137: 2831–2834
Modlin RL, Gersuk GM, Nelson EE, Pattengale PK, Gunter JR, Chen L, Cooper CL, Bloom BR, Rea TH (1986b) T-lymphocyte clones from leprosy skin lesions. Lepr Rev 57 [Suppl 2]: 143–147
Modlin RL, Mehra V, Jordan R, Bloom BR, Rea TH (1986c) In situ and in vitro characterization of the cellular immune response in erythema nodosum leprosum. J Immunol 136: 883–886
Modlin RL, Kato H, Mehra V, Nelson EE, Xue-dong F, Rea TH Pattengale PK, Bloom BR (1986d) Genetically restricted suppressor T-cell clones derived from lepromatous leprosy lesions. Nature 322: 459–461
Modlin RL, Brenner MB, Krangel MS, Duby AD, Bloom BR (1987) T-cell receptors of human suppressor cells. Nature 329: 541–545
Modlin RL, Melancon-Kaplan J, Young SMM, Pirmez C, Kino H, Convit J, Rea TH, Bloom BR (1988) Learning from lesions: patterns of tissue inflammation in leprosy. Proc Natl Acad Sci USA 85: 1213–1217

Modlin RL, Pirmez C, Hofman FM, Torigian V, Uyemura K, Rea TH, Bloom BR Brenner MB (1989) Lymphocytes bearing antigen-specific $\gamma\delta$ T-cell receptors accumulate in human infectious disease lesions Nature 339: 544–548

Mustafa AS, Godal T (1987) BCG induced $CD4^+$ cytotoxic T cells from BCG vaccinated healthy subjects: relation between cytotoxicity and suppression in vitro. Clin Exp Immunol 69: 255–262

Narayanan RB, Bhutani LK, Sharma AK, Nath I (1983) T cell subsets in leprosy lesions: in situ characterization using monoclonal antibodies. Clin Exp Immunol 51: 421–429

Narayanan RB, Laal S, Sharma AK, Bhutani LK, Nath I (1984) Differences in predominant T cell phenotypes and distribution pattern in reactional lesions of tuberculoid and lepromatous leprosy. Clin Exp Immunol 55: 623–628

Nathan CF, Kaplan G, Levis WR, Nusrat A, Witmer MD, Sherwin SA, Job CK, Horowitz CR, Steinman RM, Cohn ZA (1986) Local and systemic effects of intradermal recombinant interferon-gamma in patients with lepromatous leprosy. N Engl J Med 315: 6–15

Nelson EE, Wong L, Uyemura K, Rea TH, Modlin RL (1987) Lepromin-induced suppressor cells in lepromatous leprosy. Cell Immunol 104: 99–104

Nilsen R, Mshana RN, Negesse Y, Menigistu G, Kana B (1986) Immunohistochemical studies of leprous neuritis. Lepr Rev 57 [Suppl 2]: 177–187

Ottenhoff THM, Elferink DG, Klaster PR, de Vries RRP (1986) Cloned suppressor T cells from a lepromatous leprosy patient suppress *Mycobacterium leprae* reactive helper T cells. Nature 322: 462–464

Ridley DS, Jopling WH (1966) Classification of leprosy according to immunity. A five-group system. Int J Leprosy 34: 255–273

Rook GAW, Steele J, Fraher L, Barker S, Karmali R, O'Riordan J (1986) Vitamin D_3, gamma interferon, and control of proliferation of *Mycobacterium tuberculosis* by human monocytes. Immunology 57: 159–163

Salgame P, Modlin R, Bloom BR (1989) On the mechanism of human T cell Suppression International Immunol 1: 121–129

Sanders ME, Makgoba MW, Shaw S (1988) Human naive and memory T cells: reinterpretation of helper-inducer and suppressor-inducer subsets. Immunol Today 9: 195–199

Sarno EN, Kaplan G, Alvaranga F, Nogueira N, Porto JA, Cohn ZA (1984) Effect of treatment on the cellular composition of cutaneous lesions in leprosy patients. Int J Leprosy 52: 496–500

van Voorhis WC, Kaplan G, Sarno EN, Horwitz MA, Steinman RM, Levis WR, Nogueira N, Hair LS, Gattass CR, Arrick BA, Cohn ZA (1982) The cutaneous infiltrates of leprosy: cellular characteristics and the predominant T-cell phenotypes. N Engl J Med 307: 1593–1597

Wallach D, Flageul B, Bach MA, Cottenot F (1984) The cellular content of dermal leprous granulomas: an immuno-histological approach. Int J Leprosy 52: 318–326

Yamada H, Martin PJ, Bean MA,Braun MP, Beatty PG, Sadamoto K, Hansen JA (1985) Monoclonal antibody 9.3 and anti-CD11 antibodies define reciprocal subsets of lymphocytes. Eur J Immunol 15: 1164–1168

Young DB, Lamb JR (1986) T lymphocytes respond to solid-phase antigen: a novel approach to the molecular analysis of cellular immunity. Immunology 59: 167–171

Antigen Reactivity and Autoreactivity: Two Sides of the Cellular Immune Response Induced by Mycobacteria

T. H. M. OTTENHOFF and R. R. P. DE VRIES

1 Introduction

Bacteria possess a pronounced, universal philosophy: to multiply and survive in the best attainable environment—the living host. The dialectic and systematic process through which bacteria pursue this philosophy is one of continuous change. This process of change is directed not by logic but by chance; bacteria generate an endless series of random variants, only some of which are positively selected because they result in better adaptation to the host. Not smart enough to make the selection themselves, they leave this to their environment. The result is ever better adapted micro-organisms that successfully infect at least part of the host population, multiply and exist.

From the point of view of the host, however, these adapted micro-organisms are a continuous threat. Therefore the host tries to recognize and eliminate potentially pathogenic microbes. Neither any human being nor any human immune system, however, is perfect. The repertoire of choices and diversities is not unlimited, and it is exactly this human weakness that bacteria in the end trace and exploit: the better host-adapted parasite penetrates into they grey and ill-defined areas between nonself- (i.e., protective), non- and self-reactivity, for example, by evading immune recognition per se, by inducing nonresponsiveness or by mimicking self antigens. Each of these possibilities are exploited by *Mycobacterium leprae*, the causative organism of leprosy and from this point of view one of the most intelligent microbes in the bacterial world.

In this chapter we focus on T cell responses induced by *M. leprae*, with an emphasis on cytotoxic T cells.

* This research was supported by the Immunology of Leprosy (IMMLEP) component of the UNDP/World Bank/WHO Special Programme For Research and Training in Tropical Diseases, the Netherlands Leprosy Relief Association (NSL), the Dutch Foundation for Medical and Health Research (MEDIGON, grant number 900-509-099) and the J.A. Cohen Institute for Radiopathology and Radiation Protection

Department of Immunohaematology and Blood Bank, University Hospital, PO Box 9600, 2300 RC Leiden, the Netherlands

Current Topics in Microbiology and Immunology, Vol. 155

2 Mycobacteria Induce Antigen-Specific and Antigen-Nonspecific Cytotoxic Cells

The cell-mediated immune response is of crucial importance in the protection against facultative intracellular bacteria such as mycobacteria (Bloom and Godal 1983; Hahn and Kaufmann 1981). So far, attempts to define the type and function of the cells involved in the cellular immune response to such bacteria have focussed mainly on antigen-specific $CD4^+CD8^-$ proliferative helper T cells. Upon recognition of antigen plus major histocompatibility comples (MHC) class II on the surface of monocytes/macrophages, Th cells secrete effector lymphokines such as interferon-γ that trigger mononuclear phagocytes to inhibit the growth of intracellular mycobacteria. But recently the possibility was suggested that immunity against mycobacterial infections could also involve the lysis of cells infected by the bacteria. Since pathogenic mycobacteria such as *M. tuberculosis* and *M. leprae* invade cells of the monocytes/macrophage series, the antigen-specific lysis of such cells may be of importance not only for the elimination of the bacterial reservoir but also for the induction of immunopathological lesions that are prevalent in tuberculosis and leprosy.

The involvment of cytotoxic cells in experimental mycobacterial infections has been supported by a number of observations. Firstly, $CD4^+$ mycobacterial antigen-specific T-lymphocytes have been shown to be capable not only of secreting macrophage-activating factors, but also of lysing macrophages infected with *M. tuberculosis* (Kaufmann and Flech 1986; Mustafa and Godal 1987). Secondly, during immunization with intracellular micro-organisms not only $CD4^+CD8^-$ but also $CD8^+CD4^-$ antigen-specific T-lymphocytes are induced (Pedrazzini et al. 1987; DeLibero and Kaufmann 1986; Chiplunkar et al. 1986; Adu et al. 1983; Pavlov et al. 1982; Orme and Collins 1984; Orme 1987; Bishop and Hinrichs 1987). The latter T cells are able to lyse antigen-infected target cells in a MHC class I restricted as well as nonrestricted fashion in vitro (DeLibero and Kaufmann 1986; Chiplunkar et al. 1986). In vivo depletion and adoptive transfer studies have established that also $CD4^-CD8^+$ T-lymphocytes confer resistance to *M. tuberculosis* (Bishop and Hinrichs 1987) and a variety of other intracellular parasites (Pedrazzini et al. 1987; Adu et al. 1983; Pavlov et al. 1982; Orme and Collins 1984, Bishop and Hinrichs 1987). Thirdly, in addition to antigen-specific T-lymphocytes, also natural killer (NK) and/or activated killer (AK) cells have been implicated in the resistance to certain intracellular parasites (Petkus and Baum 1987). Mycobacteria in particular are known to be potent activators of NK cell activity (Eugui and Allison 1987).

We therefore have investigated the possible role of cytolytic effector cells in the cellular response to mycobacterial antigens. Table 1 summarizes in brief experiments performed at the Armauer Hansen Research Institute (Birhane Kaleab et al., manuscripts submitted). Antigen-pulsed or -nonpulsed, ^{51}Cr-labelled adherent cells of peripheral blood mononuclear cells were used as target cells for 7-day antigen-educated effector cells obtained from mycobacterial antigen-responsive donors, either healthy *M. leprae* exposed individuals or leprosy patients. The percentage ^{51}Cr release was determined after 12–15 hours as described in Birhane

Table 1. Cytolytic effector cells in the cellular response to mycobacterial antigens

Effector cells stimulated with	Lysis of autologous macrophages pulsed with					Lysis of K562/Daudi
	BCG	PPD	*M. leprae*	Tetanus toxoid	No antigen	
BCG	+ + +	+ + +	+ +	+	+	+ + +
PPD	+ + +	+ + +	ND	+	+	+ + +
M. leprae	+ + +	ND	+ + +	+	+	+ + +
No antigen	–	–	–	–	–	–

KALEAB et al. (submitted for publication). Bacille Calmette-Guérin (BCG), purified protein derivative (PPD) of *M. tuberculosis* and *M. leprae*-stimulated effector cells efficiently lysed autologous adherent cells that had been pulsed with the homologous antigen. Cross-reactivity between the different mycobacterial antigens was apparent, as expected. Furthermore, antigen-stimulated effector cells significantly lysed tumour target cells such as the K562 and Daudi lines and, interestingly, also macrophages that had not been pulsed with antigen, albeit much less efficiently than the corresponding pulsed target macrophages.

The MHC restriction and membrane phenotype of antigen-induced cytolytic effector cells varied with the type of antigen used (see Table 2) as well as between different donors. BCG- and PPD- and *M. leprae*-educated cytotoxic cells all displayed specific lysis of antigen-pulsed autologous but not antigen-pulsed allogeneic (HLA-mismatched) macrophages. The active population of the PPD-stimulated specific effector cells consisted almost entirely of $CD4^+CD8^-$HLA-DR restricted T cells, as determined by depletion experiments in which the reciprocal subsets were taken away with monoclonal antibody coated magnetic beads and by blocking experiments with HLA-specific monoclonal antibodies. The picture for BCG- and *M. leprae*-stimulated effector cells is more complex, as indicated in Table 2, with inter-individually varying contributions of $CD4^+$ and $CD8^+$ and of class II and class I restricted cytolytic effector cells. Those observations convinced us of the importance of cytotoxic effector cells in the immune response to mycobacterial antigens. Another series of experiments showed that these cytotoxic cells were not only able to lyse macrophages but also to inhibit the outgrowth of live, intracellularly located mycobacteria (D.S. KUMARARATNE, BIRHANE KALEAB, R. KIESSLING, P. CONVERSE and T. OTTENHOFF, unpublished observations). The implication of these results is that cytotoxic cells may be pivotal effector cells in

Table 2. MHC restriction and membrane phenotype of antigen-induced effector cells

Effector cells stimulated with	Lysis of				Specificity of MHC-directed MAb that inhibit antigen-dependent lysis of macrophages	Active cytotoxic T-cell subset as determined by depletion experiments
	Autologous macrophages pulsed with		Allogeneic macrophages pulsed with			
	antigen	no antigen	antigen	no antigen		
BCG	+ + +	+	+	+	Class II and /or, Class I	CD4, CD8
PPD	+ + +	+	+	+	Class II	CD4
M. leprae	+ + +	+	+	+	Class I and/or Class II	CD8, CD4

the protection against mycobacterial infections. If this is indeed true, it follows that definition of the microbial components that trigger such cells would be an important step towards the development of protective mycobacterial subunit vaccines (BLOOM and GODAL 1983).

In search of such antigens, we, like many other groups, have recently studied the recombinant 65-kDa heat-shock protein of *M. bovis* BCG/*M. tuberculosis*. One reason for doing this was a practical one, namely its availability on a large scale through the stimulating efforts of the Immunology of Leprosy and Immunology of Tuberculosis programmes.

The more important reason behind its being available, of course, is its immunological importance: the 65-kDa antigen expresses multiple epitopes that are recognized by antibodies of immunized animals (YOUNG et al. 1987; THOLE et al. 1988; ENGERS et al. 1986; MEHRA et al. 1986; BUCHANAN et al. 1987; SHINNICK et al. 1987; HUSSON and YOUNG 1987; DE BRUYN et al. 1987). Also, the 65-kDa mycobacterial antigen appears to be an important structure for T-cell recognition in mice (KAUFMANN et al. 1987). In humans, $CD4^+$ proliferative helper T-cell clones, selected for reactivity to *M. leprae* to *M. tuberculosis*, have been found to recognize frequently the r65-kDa mycobacterial heat-shock protein or synthetic peptides of the molecule (YOUNG et al. 1987; THOLE et al. 1988; EMMRICH et al. 1986; LAMB et al. 1987; OFTUNG et al. 1987; VAN SCHOOTEN et al., in press). Little was known, however, about the possible immunodominance of the 65-kDa antigen in the triggering of unselected polyclonal, rather than monoclonal, selected T cells.

Besides its immunodominance, another extremely interesting characteristic of the 65-kDa antigen is its being a heat-shock protein (YOUNG et al. 1988). The ubiquitous nature–and thus probably function–of such proteins in different species points to a highly conserved structure. Indeed, the recent comparison of the sequences of the 65-kDa mycobacterial heat-shock protein and its human counterpart strongly support this notion (R.A. YOUNG, personal communication). The paradox of, on the one hand, high immunogenicity and, on the other, high homology with self-structures makes the 65-kDa molecule an intriguing antigen to study. The scene for immunity towards the 65-kDa heat-shock protein must be enacted at the boundaries of protection, self-reactivity and tolerance.

In the grey and shady areas between these entities, seemingly strict boundaries could sometimes be blurred, with the result of either autoreactivity or lack of protective immunity.

3 The Mycobacterial r65kDa Heat-Shock Antigen Induces Antigen-Specific as well as Antigen-Nonspecific Cytotoxic Cells

For these reasons we studied the role of the r65-kDa antigen of *M. bovis* BCG/*M. tuberculosis* in the polyclonal human immune response. A total of 58, mostly Ethiopian individuals (including healthy and leprosy-affected ones) were randomly

Table 3. Proliferative responses of PBMC from different individuals to *M.* bovis BCG, *M.* leprae and the recombinant 65-kDa of BCG protein. (From OTTENHOFF et al. 1988)

Case no.	Clinical diagnosis	BCG/PPD	65-kDa protein	*M. leprae*	Control
1	Normal	145204 ± 8733	53710 ± 1989	51493 ± 4797	821 ± 607
2	Normal	162243 ± 19895	12229 ± 3674	66261 ± 6333	2208 ± 306
3	Normal	60607 ± 11584	9989 ± 3497	19507 ± 2381	540 ± 122
4	Normal	172745 ± 14839	20585 ± 5305	ND	1116 ± 453
5	Normal	140741 ± 4314	5906 ± 6	8093 ± 2955	1633 ± 466
6	BT	55735 ± 7758	10504 ± 2011	56140 ± 11884	2369 ± 812
7	BT	61260 ± 11991	5796 ± 508	23711 ± 4057	1834 ± 811
8	BT	53524 ± 22786	22535 ± 3286	5807 ± 1264	2863 ± 851
9	LL	59357 ± 12137	21901 ± 5175	955 ± 98	1202 ± 224

BT, Borderline tuberculoid leprosy; LL, lepromatous leprosy.
The results are expressed as mean cpm ± SEM of [^{3}H] thymidine incorporation by triplicate cultures of 2×10^5 PBMC each. Results are shown only for the 9 out of 47 (21 healthy contacts, 13 BT, and 13 LL patients) BCG-responsive individuals that responded to the recombinant 65-kDa protein.

tested in standard lymphocyte proliferative (LTT) assays against BCG, *M. leprae* and the r65-kDa of BCG antigen. Of the 47 BCG responders (cpm > 5000), 9(± 20%) also responded to the r65-kDa antigen, as shown in Table 3 (OTTENHOFF et al. 1988). Earlier (BIRHANE KALEAB et al., manuscripts submitted) we had noted a highly significant correlation between the percentage of specific lysis of antigen-pulsed monocytes by antigen-educated effector cells and the proliferative response of the individual to the same antigen. Thus all LTT responders yielded efficient killer cells to monocytes pulsed with the specific antigen, while poor LTT responders mediated little if any cytotoxicity.

This correlation also appeared to hold true for the r65-kDa antigen. PPD- or BCG-stimulated effector cells from 65-kDa responsive donors efficiently lysed PPD-pulsed, and to a much lower extent, nonpulsed or tetanus toxoid pulsed autologous macrophages in a dose-dependent manner (Table 4). PPD-induced effector cells of r65-kDa (LTT) responsive donors also lysed r65-kDa pulsed monocytes efficiently. PPD-stimulated effector cells of r65-kDa LTT nonresponders lysed PPD-pulsed but not r65-kDa pulsed monocytes (not shown). The r65-kDa protein of BCG therefore appears to be an important target molecule for PPD- or BCG-stimulated cytotoxic effector cells of r65-kDa LTT-responsive donors.

To investigate whether the r65-kDa heat-shock protein of BCG also was immunodominant at the precursor rather than at the effector level, we raised r65-kDa stimulated effector cells from LTT-responsive donors. These effector cells efficiently lysed r65-kDa pulsed monocytes and, importantly, also PPD-pulsed monocytes. Nonpulsed or irrelevant antigen-pulsed monocytes were lysed to a lower extent than PPD-pulsed or r65-kDa pulsed ones, but r65-kDa induced effector cells lysed nonpulsed monocytes more efficiently than did PPD- or BCG-induced cytotoxic cells. Antigen-pulsed and nonpulsed target cells were equally sensitive to lysis by lymphokine-activated killer (LAK) cells, ruling out the possibility that (mycobacterial) antigen pulsing in itself would render monocytes more susceptible to nonspecific lysis by effector cells.

The r65-kDa heat-shock protein of BCG is thus an efficient stimulatory

Table 4. Antigen-specific and antigen-nonspecific lysis of macrophage targets by BCG/PPD or recombinant 65-kD-HSP of BCG-stimulated cytotoxic effector lymphocytes

Individual	Stimulating antigen	E/T ratio	PPD	Percent specific lysis of macrophages pulsed with		
				65-kD HSP BCG	Tetanus toxoid	No antigen
1	PPD	40:1	69	62	ND	29
		12:1	67	58	ND	22
		4:1	57	52	ND	14
		40:1	50	63	ND	41
	r65-kD BCG	12:1	60	61	ND	35
		4:1	56	57	ND	25
2	PPD	50:1	45	29	21	20
		15:1	57	22	19	12
		5:1	38	16	0	5
		25:1	33	37	23	20
	r65-kD BCG	8:1	19	26	12	10
		2:1	9	10	2	1
3	PPD	25:1	58	32	ND	13
		8:1	42	26	ND	8
		2:1	25	12	ND	2
	r65-kD BCG	25:1	42	36	ND	27
		8:1	34	29	ND	15
		2:1	25	19	ND	9
	rIL-2	25:1	12	15	ND	15
		8:1	16	7	ND	12
		2:1	5	2	ND	3

E/T ratio, ratio of effector cells to target cells; HSP, heat-shock protein

molecule for precursors of cytotoxic effector cells that specifically lyse PPD-pulsed and r65-kDa pulsed monocytes but also strongly lyse monocytes in the absence of antigen.

Both PPD and r65-kDa triggered effector cells consisted mainly of $CD4^+$ T cells ($CD3^+$/$CD5^+$) (Ottenhoff et al. 1988; Birhane Kaleab et al. submitted). A remarkable difference, however, was the much higher expression of the leu-19(HNK-1) markers by r65-kDa stimulated effector cells as compared to PPD-raised ones (not shown). The leu-19 marker is found on NK cells and activated T cells. In parallel with the higher leu-19 expression, there also was a higher expression of CD8 marker among r65-kDa heat-shock rotein induced effector cells. In order to determine the phenotype of the actual r65-kDa of BCG-induced effector cytotoxic T cells, depletion experiments were performed using monoclonal antibody coated magnetic beads. Only depletion of $CD4^+$ or $CD5^+$ but not $CD8^+$ or leu-19^+ (or control) cells from the r65-kDa stimulated effector population significantly reduced or abolished lysis of r65-kDa pulsed monocytes (not shown). Antigen dependent lysis by r65-kDa effectors was HLA-DR restricted. Antigen-specific lysis of antigen-pulsed monocytes by r65-kDa effector cells thus is mediated by a CD3/5^+, $CD4^+$, $CD8^-$, leu-19^- T-cell population.

Table 5. Cytotoxicity of effector cells to K562 and Daudi tumour cells by mycobacterial antigen induced cytotoxic effector cells

	Percent specific lysis of					
	K562			Daudi		
Effector cells Stimulated with:	PPD	r65-kD	No antigen	PPD	r65-kDa	No antigen
E/T ratio						
35:1	51	66	1	55	66	9
12:1	17	29	3	28	40	4
4:1	8	20	1	7	14	0
1:1	5	4	0	0	4	0

Because, however, the r65-kDa heat-shock protein of BCG stimulated effector cells efficiently lysed nonpulsed monocytes and strongly expressed the leu-19 antigen, we tested whether these effectors also were cytotoxic to K562 (the conventional NK target) and Daudi (NK-resistant but AK-sensitive target) tumour cells. As shown in Table 5, PPD and r65-kDa stimulated effector cells lysed both target cells, indicating that they indeed display NK-like and AK activity. The fact that r65-kDa educated effector cells display such relatively strong nonspecific cytotoxicity may be an important factor with regard to the possible pathological role of this heat-shock protein in autoimmunity (e.g., VAN EDEN et al. 1988; RES et al. 1988); nonspecific lysis of tissue macrophages and other autologous targets may lead to tissue damage, which is indeed a prominent feature of mycobacterioses such as tuberculoid leprosy and tuberculosis.

It is not yet clear whether the effector cells responsible for nonspecific lysis of monocytes are different from those active in specific killing, or whether both types of activities are activated through the same determinants on the 65-kDa protein. It will be important to try to dissociate the r65-kDa determinants that induce specific versus nonspecific cytotoxicity since, if possible, only the former determinants could then be selected for in vivo (vaccine) use. Another possibility, however, is that r65-kDa mycobacterial heat-shock protein induced cytotoxic T cells cross-react with the human 65-kDa homologue that is probably expressed during inflammatory reactions by monocytes (POLLA 1988; J.D.A VAN EMBDEN, personal communication). In such a case, the advantages of immunogenicity would have to be weighed against the disadvantages of autoreactivity induced by the r65-kDa heat-shock protein, although it cannot be excluded that autoreactivity is an essential mechanism in clearing intracellularly located mycobacterial reservoirs from the body.

An intriguing question that remains unanswered is why the r65-kDa antigen is such an important antigen for cytotoxic T cells. An answer may lie in its identity as a heat-shock protein, able to bind certain other proteins. If the 65-kDa heat-shock protein of BCG is able to be translocated across membranes and to bind easily to other proteins, it could have a quantitatively privileged access to the endosomal/lysosomal processing pathway and to carrier HLA molecules.

4 Mycobacterial r65-kDa Heat-Shock Protein reactive T cell clones

To answer these questions, we have cloned mycobacterium-reactive T-cell clones. Most clones were raised from the peripheral blood of leprosy patients using a protocol in which *M. leprae* was used to select for mycobacterium reactive cells (VAN SCHOOTEN et al. 1988; HAANEN et al. 1986; OTTENHOFF et al. 1986a, b). By far the majority of the clones thus obtained were $CD4^{+}CD8^{-}$. They proliferated and produced interferon-γ to *M. leprae* or other mycobacterial antigens presented by HLA class II molecules, nearly always HLA-DR (OTTENHOFF et al. 1986c).

In accord with previous reports (EMMRICH et al. 1986; OFTUNG et al. 1987; DE VRIES et al. 1986) a remarkably high percentage (20%–30%) of these clones were reactive with the 65-kDa protein (VAN SCHOOTEN et al. 1988). Mapping of the epitopes on the mycobacterial 65-kDa recognized by these clones was performed using deletion mutants of the 65-kDa gene and synthetic peptides (THOLE et al. 1988; LAMB et al. 1987; VAN SCHOOTEN et al., in press). Figure 1 shows a map of most of the T-cell epitopes defined on the mycobacterial r65-kDa protein and the clear HLA-DR Ir gene control of the response to these epitopes. Thus far each epitope is presented by only one particular HLA-DR allele (VAN SCHOOTEN et al., in press).

From the foregoing it is clear that one of the key questions is whether T cells reactive with the mycobacterial 65-kDa protein cross-react with the human homologue. This has indeed been observed (J.R. LAMB et al., 1989). We are presently also investigating this issue, both in infectious and in auto immune diseases.

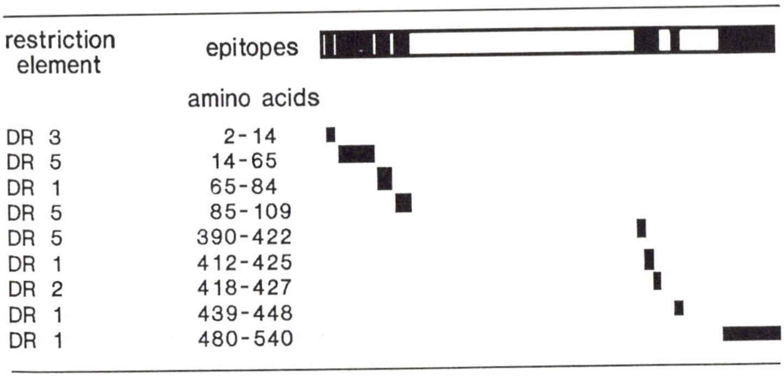

restriction element
epitopes
amino acids
DR 3
2-14
DR 5
14-65
DR 1
65-84
DR 5
85-109
DR 5
390-422
DR 1
412-425
DR 2
418-427
DR 1
439-448
DR 1
480-540

Fig. 1. The 65-kDa mycobacterial protein: T-cell epitopes and HLA-DR IR gene control. T-cell epitope map of the 65-kDa mycobacterial protein. The restriction element of 65-kDa reactive T-cell clones and lines was established with the use of inhibition studies with anti-HLA monoclonal antibodies and a panel of HLA-typed allogeneic antigen-presenting cells. The T-cell epitopes were mapped using deletion mutants of the 65-kDa gene and synthetic peptides (THOLE et al. 1988; LAMB et al. 1987; VAN SCHOOTEN et al., submitted for publication)

Acknowledgements. The majority of the work presented here was done in the Armauer Hansen Research Institute, Addis Ababa, Ethiopia, founded by the Norwegian and Swedish Save the Children Funds and now supported by the Swedish and Norwegian development agencies; it is affiliated with the All Africa Leprosy Rehabilitation and Training Centre (ALERT), Addis Ababa, Ethiopia. The last part of the work reviewed here was performed at the Department of Immunohaetology and Blood Bank, University Hospital, Leiden, the Netherlands.

References

Adu HO, Curtis J, Turk JL (1983) The resistance of C57BL/6 mice to subcutaneous infection with *Mycobacterium lepraemurium* is dependent on both T cells and other cells of bone marrow origin. Cell Immunol 78: 249

Birhane Kaleab R, Kiessling P, Converse G, Tadesse, Ottenhoff T a Mycobacterial antigen induced cytotoxic cells. I. *Mycobacterium bovis* BCG and *M. leprae* induce antigen specific cytotoxic T cells as well as antigen non-specific killer cells that lyse macrophages of healthy exposed individuals and leprosy patients in vitro. (submitted for publication)

Birhane Kaleab R, Kiessling M, Rottenberg P, Converse A, Wondimu , Ottenhoff T b Mycobacterial antigen induced cytotoxic cells. II. Membrane- and HLA-restriction-phenotype of *Mycobacterium bovis* BCG and *M. leprae* induced cytotoxic cells (Manuscript in preparation)

Birhane Kaleab R, Kiessling JDA, van Embden JER, Thole DS, Kumararatne P, Pisa A, Wondimu , Ottenhoff THM c Induction of antigen specific $CD4^+$ HLA-DR restricted cytotoxic T lymphocytes as well as nonspecific nonrestricted killer cells by the recombinant mycobacterial 65 kilodalton heat shock protein (submitted for publication)

Bishop DK, Hinrichs DJ (1987) Adoptive transfer of immunity to *Listeria monocytogenes*. The influence of in vitro stimulation on lymphocyte subset requirements. J Immunol 139: 2005

Bloom BR, Godal T (1983) Selective primary health care: strategies for control of disease in the developing world. V. Leprosy. Rev Infect Dis 5: 765

Buchanan TM, Nomaguchi H, Anderson DC, Young RA, Gillis TP, Britton WJ, Ivanyi J, Kolk AHJ, Closs O, Bloom BR, Mehra V (1987) Characterization of antibody reactive epitopes on the 65-kilodalton protein of *Mycobacterium leprae*. Infect Immun 55: 1000

Chiplunkar S, De Libero G, Kaufmann SHE (1986) *Mycobacterium leprae* specific $lyt2^+$ T lymphocytes with cytolytic activity. Infect Immun 54: 793

De Bruyn J, Bosmans R, Turneer M, Weckx M, Nyabenda J, van Vooren JP, Falmagne P, Wilker HG, Harboe M (1987) Purification, partial characterization and identification of a skin reactive protein antigen of *Mycobacterium bovis* BCG. Infect Immun 55: 245

De Libero G, Kaufmann SHE (1986) Antigen specific $lyt2^+$ cytolytic T lymphocytes from mice infected with the intracellular bacterium *Listeria monocytogenes*. J Immunol 137: 2688

De Vries RRP, Ottenhoff THM, LI Shuguang, Young RA (1986) HLA class II-restricted helper and suppressor clones reactive with *Mycobacterium leprae*. Lepr Rev 57: 113

Emmrich F, Thole J, van Embden J, Kaufmann SHE (1986) A recombinant 64kD protein of *Mycobacterium bovis* BCG specifically stimulates human T4 clones reactive to mycobacterial antigens. J Exp Med 163 1024

Engers HD, Abe M, Bloom BR, Britton W, Buchanan TM, Khanolkar SK, Young DB, Closs O, Gillis T, Harboe M, Ivanyi J, Kolk AHJ, Shepard CC (1985) Results of a World Health Organization-sponsored workshop on monoclonal antibodies to *Mycobacterium leprae*. Infect Immun 48: 603

Eugui E.M, Allison AC (1987) Activation of natural killer cells and its possible role in immunity to intracellular parasites. In: Torrigiani G, Bell R (eds) Immunological recognition and effector mechanisms in infectious diseases. Schwabe, Basel p 161

Haanen JBAG, Ottenhoff THM, Voordouw A, Elferink BG, Klatser PR, Spits H, de Vries RRP (1986) HLA class II restricted *Mycobacterium leprae* reactive T cell clones from leprosy patients established with a minimal requirement for autologous mononuclear cells. Scand J Immunol 23: 101

Hahn H, Kaufmann SHE (1981) The role of cell-mediated immunity in bacterial infections. Rev Infect Dis 3: 1221

Husson RN, Young RA (1987) Genes for the major protein antigens of *Mycobacterium tuberculosis*: the etiologic agents of tuberculosis and leprosy share an immunodominant antigen. Proc Natl Acad Sci USA 84: 1679

Kaufmann SHE, Flesch I (1986) Function and antigen recognition pattern of L3T4$^+$ T-cell clones from *Mycobacterium tuberculosis* immune mice. Infect Immun 54: 291

Kaufmann SHE, Vath U, Thole JER, van Embden JDA, Emmrich F (1987) Enumeration of T cells reactive with *Mycobacterium tuberculosis* organisms and specific for the recombinant mycobacterial 64kDa protein. Eur J Immunol 17: 531

Lamb JR, Ivanyi J, Rees ADM, Rothbard JB, Howland K, Young RA, Young DB (1987) Mapping of T cell epitopes using recombinant antigens and synthetic peptides. EMBO J 6: 1245

Lamb JR, Bal V, Mendez-Samperio P, Mehlert A, So A, Rothbard J, Jindal S, Young RA and Young DB (1989) Stress proteins may provide a link between the immune response to infection and autoimmunity. Internat. Immunol. 1: 191

Mehra V, Sweetser D, Young RA (1986) Efficient mapping of protein antigenic determinants. Proc natl Acad Sci USA 83: 7013

Mustafa AS, Godal T (1987) BCG induced CD4$^+$ cytotoxic T cells from BCG vaccinated healthy subjects: relation between cytotoxicity and suppression in vitro. Clin Exp Immunol 69: 255

Oftung F, Mustafa AS, Husson RN, Young RA, Godal T (1987) Human T-cell clones recognize two abundant *M. tuberculosis* antigens expressed in *E. coli.* J Immunol 138: 927

Orme IM (1987) The kinetics of emergence and loss of mediator T lymphocytes acquired in response to infection with *Mycobacterium tuberculosis.* J Immunol 138: 293

Orme IM, Collins FM (1984) Adoptive protection of the *Mycobacterium tuberculosis* infected lung. Dissociation between cells that passively transfer protective immunity and those that transfer delayed type hypersensitivity to tuberculin. Cell Immunol 84: 113

Ottenhoff THM, Klatser PR, Ivanyi J, Elferink BG, de Wit MYL, de Vries RRP (1986a) *Mycobacterium leprae*-specific protein antigens defined by cloned human helper T cells. Nature 319: 66

Ottenhoff THM, Elferink BG, Klatser PR, de Vries RRP (1986b) Cloned suppressor T cells from a lepromatous leprosy patient suppress *Mycobacterium leprae*-reactive helper T cells. Nature 322: 462

Ottenhoff THM, Neuteboom S, Elferink BG, de Vries RRP (1986c) Molecular localisation and polymorphism of HLA class II restriction determinants defined by *Mycobacterium leprae*-reactive helper T cell clones from leprosy patients. J Exp Med 164: 1923

Ottenhoff THM, Birhane Kaleab R, van Embden JDA, Thole JER, Kiessling R (1988) The recombinant 65 kilodalton heat shock protein of *Mycobacterium bovis* BCG/*M. tuberculosis* is a target molecule for CD4$^+$ cytotoxic T lymphocytes that lyse human monocytes. J Exp Med 168: 1947

Pavlov H, Hogarth M, McKenzie IFC, Cheers C (1982) In vivo and In vitro effects of monoclonal antibody to Ly antigens or immunity to infection. Cell Immunol 71: 127

Pedrazzini T, Hug K, Louis JA (1987) Importance of L3T4$^+$ and Lyt2$^+$ cells in the immunologic control of infection with *Mycobacterium bovis* strain *basillus Calmette Guerin* in mice. Assessment by elimination of T cell subsets in vivo. J Immunol 138: 2032

Petkus AF, Baum LL (1987) Natural killer cell inhibition of young spherules and endospores of *Coccidioides immitis.* J Immunol 139: 3107

Polla BS (1988) A role for heat shock proteins in inflammation? Immunol Today 9: 134

Res P, Schaar CG, Breedveld FC, van Eden W, van Embden JDA, Cohen IR, de Vries RRP (1988) Synovial fluid T cell reactivity against 65kD heat shock protein of mycobacteria in early chronic arthritis. Lancet ii: 479

Shinnick TM, Sweetser D, Thole JER, van Embden JDA, Young RA (1987) The etiologic agents of leprosy and tuberculosis share an immunoreactive protein antigen with the vaccine strain *Mycobacterium bovis* BCG. Infect Immun 55: 1932

Thole JER, van Schooten WCA, Keulen WJ, Hermans PWM, Janson AAM, de Vries RRP, Kolk AHJ, van Embden JDA (1988) Use of recombinant antigens expressed in *Escherichia coli* K-12 to map B cell and T cell epitopes on the immunodominant 65 kilodalton protein of *Mycobacterium bovis* BCG. Infect Immun 56: 1633

van Eden W, Thole JER, van der Zee R, Noordzy A, van Embden JDA, Hensen EJ, Cohen IR (1988) Cloning of the mycobacterial epitope recognized by T lymphocytes in adjuvant arthritis. Nature 331: 171

Van Schooten WCA, Ottenhoff THM, Klatser PR, Thole JER, de Vries RRP, Kolk AHJ (1988) T cell epitopes on the 36K and 65K *Mycobacterium leprae* antigens defined by human T cell clones. Eur J Immunol 18: 849

Van Schooten WCA, Elferink DG, van Embden J, Anderson DC, de Vries RRP DR3 restricted T cells from different HLA-DR3 positive individuals recognize the same peptide aa2-12 of the mycobacterial 65kDa heat shock protein. Eur J Immunol, in press

Young DB, Ivanyi J, Cox JH, Lamb JR (1987) The 65kD antigen of mycobacteria—a common bacterial protein? Immunol Today 8:215

Young D, Lathigra R, Hendrix R, Sweetser D, Young RA (1988) Stress proteins are immune targets in leprosy and tuberculosis. Proc Natl Acad Sci USA 85:4267

Antigens and Carriers

T-Cells, Stress Proteins, and Pathogenesis of Mycobacterial Infections*

S. H. E. Kaufmann, B. Schoel, A. Wand-Württenberger, U. Steinhoff, M. E. Munk, and T. Koga

1 Introduction

When a microbial pathogen meets a mammalian organism, different kinds of relationship may evolve. Exotoxin-producing pathogens can harm the host in a dramatic way without becoming too involved themselves. Purulent bacteria colonize extracellular niches from which they can cause acute-type diseases. In both cases, humoral immunity has a profound effect, and normally either type of pathogen is rapidly eliminated once it is taken up by professional phagocytes. So-called intracellular pathogens establish a lifestyle inside host cells, and many of them survive within macrophages at least for some time. Bacteria of this group include *Mycobacterium tuberculosis*, *M. bovis*, *M. leprae*, *Salmonella typhi*, *Legionella pneumophila*, and *Listeria monocytogenes*—the etiologic agents of tuberculosis, leprosy, typhoid fever, Legionnaire's disease, and listeriosis, respectively. Although macrophages provide a major habitat for these microorganisms, other host cells can be affected as well, with *M. leprae*-infected Schwann's cell providing a notable example.

The means by which phagocytes can kill intracellular pathogens are manifold and incompletely understood (Hahn and Kaufmann 1981; Kaufmann 1989). These comprise one or more of the following mechanisms: generation of reactive oxygen metabolites; changes in the phagosomal pH; low oxygen pressure; nutrient deprivation; and phagosome-lysosome fusion followed by release of lysosomal enzymes into the phagosomal compartment. Similarly manifold and incompletely understood are the means by which intracellular pathogens can evade macrophage killing (Moulder 1985; Kaufmann 1989). These include one or more of the following mechanisms: resistance to reactive oxygen metabolites or lysosomal enzymes; nutrient deprivation; pH changes; anaerobiosis; inhibition of phagosome-lysosome fusion and of reactive oxygen metabolism; and evasion from the

* Work from this laboratory received financial support to S.H.E.K. from: UNDP/World Bank/WHO Special Programme for Research and Training in Tropical Diseases; the WHO as part of its Program For Vaccine Development; Sonderforschungs-bereich 322; German Leprosy Relief Association; EEC-India Science and Technology Cooperation Program. S.H.E.K. is recipient of the A. Krupp award for young professors; T.K. is supported by the Alexander von Humboldt Foundetion; and M.E.M. is supported by the Conselho Nacional de Deservolvimento Cientifico e Tecnologico, Brazil

Department of Medical Microbiology and Immunology, University of Ulm, Albert-Einstein-Allee 11, D-7900 Ulm, FRG

Current Topics in Microbiology and Immunology, Vol. 155

phagosomal compartment into the cytoplasm. In order to benefit from their host cells, intracellular bacteria are often of low toxicity. On the other hand, the armament of many host cells is insufficient for sterile eradication of their predators. Therefore, a balance between host and pathogen becomes established which can last over long periods of time. However, this balance remains labile and depends on a multitude of factors on the part both of host and pathogen.

T cells can activate antimicrobial macrophage functions, and once T cells have been stimulated, the balance is often changed to the benefit of the host. The weaker the mechanisms allowing intracellular persistence, the more rapid may be the shift. Host cells other than macrophages are less easily activated and hence may provide longer lasting niches for intracellular microbes. In this complex of host-parasite relationships with all its peculiarities, a common feature seems to exist which can be traced down to the molecular level: the synthesis of a family of proteins through which host and pathogen attempt to avoid the insults arising from their bearing. These proteins have been termed heat-shock proteins (hsp) or stress proteins (Craig 1985; Lindquist 1986). An hsp response is not at all unique to infection; rather it represents a ubiquitous cell response to many noxious stimuli. Still, hsp seem to deserve particular attention in the field of antimicrobial immunity since in many cases they represent dominant antigens of intracellular pathogens.

2 Overview

2.1 The hsp Response

Since the discovery of an hsp response by Ritossa in 1962, this phenomenon has been observed in so many cells that it is safe to say that every cell—prokaryotic or eukaryotic—responds to stress with the synthesis of hsp (Craig 1985; Lindquist 1986). Hsp synthesis is not only induced by elevated temperature but also by a variety of environmental insults, including changes in pH, or oxygen pressure, confrontation with reactive oxygen metabolites and nutrient deprivation.

Hsp induction under sublethal conditions has been shown to protect the cell from a subsequent, more serious challenge (Gerner et al. 1976; Henle and Leeper 1976; Christman et al. 1985). Because microbial pathogens which persist in macrophages must face many of the stress stimuli mentioned above, it can be anticipated that they synthesize hsp in an attempt to protect themselves from macrophage defense. This notion is illustrated by the finding that *Salmonella typhimurium* mutants which fail to synthesize hsp in response to reactive oxygen metabolites are more susceptible to macrophage killing (Morgan et al. 1986; Fields et al. 1986). In addition, some hsp have been shown to possess ATPase activity which may allow themselves to undermine energy production of their prey and conseq-uently to inhibit energy-dependent defense mechanism (Ungewickell 1985).

In addition to the challenges mentioned above, mammalian cells synthesize hsp in response to viral infections and to physiological stimulators (Collins and

HIGHTOWER 1982; NEVINS 1982; NOTARIANNI and PRESTON 1982; KHANDJIAN and TÜRLER 1983; GARRY et al. 1983; LATHANGUE et al. 1984; LATHANGUE and LATCHMAN 1987; POLLA et al. 1987; POLLA 1988; FERRIS et al. 1988). For example, human macrophages produce hsp in response to stimulation with 1,25-dihydroxy-vitamin D_3 (POLLA et al. 1987). From this, it can be assumed that macrophages synthesize hsp to protect themselves from insults exerted by the intracellular pathogen as well as by their own antimicrobial machinery.

More recently, strong evidence has been presented that hsp fulfill several important functions in normal cells. They are involved in intracellular protein translocation, aid in the folding and unfolding of intracellular proteins, and participate in the assembly of macromolecular complexes and in membrane biogenesis (DESHAIES et al. 1988; CHIRICO et al. 1988; ELLIS 1987; PELHAM 1988; NEWPORT et al. 1988). To account for these features of hsp the term "chaperonins" has been introduced (ELLIS 1987; PELHAM 1988). These and other data are compatible with a possible role of hsp in antigen processing (VAN BUSKIRK et al. in press).

The hsp form a family of closely related proteins which have been categorized into several groups according to their size (LINDQUIST 1986). Importantly, hsp have been enormously conserved during evolution (HEMMINGSEN et al. 1988; BARDWELL and CRAIG 1984, 1987; MCMULLIN and HALLBERG 1988; JINDAL et al. 1989; YOUNG et al. 1988; GARSIA et al. 1989). An impressive example is the 65-kDa hsp of mycobacteria. This molecule is identical in *M. tuberculosis* and *M. bovis*, almost indistinguishable in *M. leprae*, and highly similar to the groEL hsp of *Escherichia coli* (YOUNG et al. 1987, 1988; SHINNICK 1987). Genes encoding similar proteins have been cloned in *Coxiella burnettii* (VODKIN and WILLIAMS 1988), *Treponema pallidum* (HINDERSSON et al. 1987), and *Borrellia burgdorferi* (HANSEN et al. 1988). Finally, it has become clear that the 65-kDa hsp is a member of the group of "common antigens" which have been identified serologically in an enormously wide range of microorganisms (THOLE et al. 1988; SHINNICK et al. 1988). It is likely that a homologue of the 65-kDa hsp is present in most, if not all bacteria man encounters naturally. From an immunological standpoint, therefore, the 65-kDa hsp represents an interesting antigen which—through the induction of an immune response to shared epitopes—could contribute to resistance against a variety of intracellular bacteria (KAUFMANN 1989).

2.2 Possible Role of the 65-kDa hsp in Acquired Resistance to Intracellular Pathogens

In the course of characterizing T-cell antigens of tubercle and leprosy bacilli T-lymphocytes with reactivity to the 65-kDa hsp have frequently been identified. In mice immunized with killed *M. tuberculosis*, about 10% of T cells with reactivity to whole *M. tuberculosis* particles recognize this particular antigen (KAUFMANN et al. 1987), and several studies have shown that it stimulates T-cell lines derived from leprosy and tuberculosis patients (EMMRICH et al. 1986; OFTUNG et al. 1987; YOUNG et al. 1987; LAMB et al. 1987; OTTENHOFF et al. 1988). Moreover, a significant number of healthy individuals possess T cells specific for the mycobacterial 65-kDa hsp (MUNK et al. 1988). Thus, the cellular immune response to the 65-kDa hsp cannot be taken as indicative for tuberculosis or leprosy, and the antigen as a whole is inappropriate for diagnosis of these diseases. Still, hsp could contribute to acquired resistance against a variety of intracellular pathogens (KAUFMANN 1989). Because of its high conservation in all microbes the 65-kDa hsp (as well as other hsp) is possibly seen by the immune system quite frequently.

When an extracellular microbe such as *E. coli* enters the circulation, it is taken up by a professional phagocyte, killed, and degraded rapidly thereafter. Hence microbes of this type should fail to supply hsp as antigens for T cells. Low-virulence microbes with the capacity to persist in host macrophages for a certain time period may, however, produce abundant quantities of hsp which could then be processed and presented to T cells. Once activated, macrophages rapidly eradicate these pathogens before clinical disease develops. Perhaps some atypical mycobacteria belong to this group of microbes which provide a constant source of hsp antigens for T-cell stimulation without causing clinical disease. When an intracellular pathogen such as *M. tuberculosis* enters the scene, infected macrophages could be recognized by cross-reactive T cells at a very early stage. Hence, T cells with specificity to shared epitopes of hsp may provide a first line of defense prior to the activation of more specific T-lymphocytes. Although they may well contribute to protection, hsp are less likely to represent a prime candidate for a vaccine that should perform better than nature already does. In fact, T cells to cross-reactive antigens of this type may have been one reason for the failure of the bacillus Calmette-Guérin vaccination trial in South India (for review see KAUFMANN 1987). The scenario outlined here, which should also be valid for other hsp, is summarized in Fig. 1.

Recently a human homologue of the mycobacterial 65-kDa hsp has been cloned (JINDAL et al. 1989). The striking homology between the mycobacterial and human 65-kDa hsp suggests that T cells with specificity to this molecule may not only contribute to antibacterial immunity but could lead to an autoimmune response as well.

3 T Cells Against Shared Self Epitopes of the 65-kDa hsp

In the following we summarize recent results obtained in our laboratory which show: (a) that autoreactive T-lymphocytes with specificity for self epitopes shared by the mycobacterial and human 65-kDa hsp exist, and (b) that these T-lymphocytes recognize stressed macrophages and Schwann's cells in the absence of exogenous antigens. It appears from our data that under physiological conditions T cells with specificity for self epitopes of the 65-kDa hsp are not activated. In certain stages of infection, however, shared peptides may be generated, and these peptides could then activate autoreactive T cells. These T cells could recognize stressed host cells and subsequently induce autoimmune reactions.

For our studies on the possible role of the 65-kDa hsp in autoimmunity large amounts of purified proteins and peptides were required. We were fortunate to have

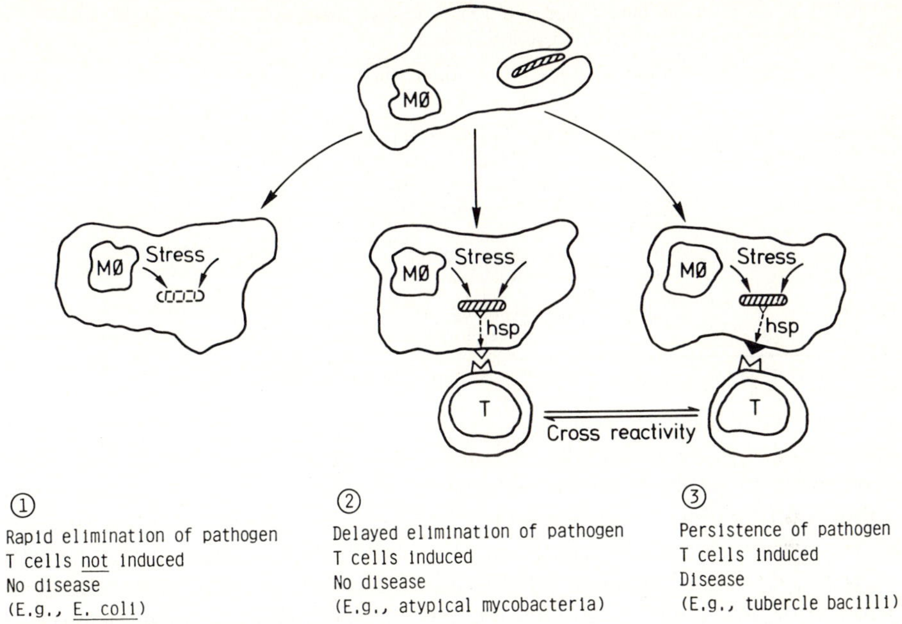

Fig. 1. Hypothetic model of how cross-reactive T cells to mycobacterial hsp could contribute to acquired resistance. Bacteria which are rapidly degraded after phagocytosis do not have sufficient time to produce hsp. Opportunistic pathogens, however, may survive for a restricted time and hence have the opportunity to produce hsp. After intracellular processing epitopes shared by a variety of microbes can be presented to T cells. These T cells recognize macrophages (*M Ø*) infected with highly virulent intracellular pathogens. Therefore these cross-reactive T cells could contribute to cross-protection at an early stage after infection

available the recombinant *E. coli* M1103 which overproduces the 65-kDa hsp of *M. bovis*/*M. tuberculosis* (THOLE et al. 1987). This clone was kindly supplied by Dr. J.D.A. van Embden. *E. coli* M1103 was grown in NYZM medium, isolated, and solubilized as described (KAUFMANN et al. 1987). The soluble material was precipitated in ammonium sulfate, and the precipitate formed between 20% and 55% saturation was purified over an anion exchange column. This material is highly enriched for the 65-kDa hsp as assessed by one- and two-dimensional gel electrophoresis. The 65-kDa hsp was denaturated in urea and, after dialysis, was digested with immobilized trypsin. Complete degradation was verified by gel filtration.

In addition, we used synthetic peptides corresponding to self epitopes of the 65-kDa hsp shared by the mycobacterial and human molecule. These peptides were synthesized and kindly supplied by Dr. S. Modrow (MODROW et al. 1989). Selection of these peptides became possible because the sequence of the human 65-kDa hsp was made known to us by Drs. R.A. Young and S. Jindal prior to publication (JINDAL et al. 1989).

When one compares the sequences of the mycobacterial and the human 65-kDa hsp, the high homology of molecules from two species so far apart is striking. Computer analysis revealed 66% similarity of the two hsp at gapweight 10 (KOGA

Table 1. Alignment of the amino acid residues of the self epitopes shared by the mycobacterial and human 65-KDa hsp

	Residual numbers	Amino acid sequence[a]
Human	109 120	AGDGTTTATVLA
M. tuberculosis	84 95	************
Human	269 289	KPLVIIAEDVDGEALSTLVLN
M. tuberculosis	243 263	***L******E********V*
		↓
Human	298 307	VAVKAPGFGD
M. tuberculosis	272 286	***************
Human	430 441	AAVEEGIVLGGG
M. tuberculosis	403 414	********A********

[a] Asterisk, identical amino acid; ↓, trypsin cleavage site within self epitopes

et al. 1989). In addition, the mycobacterial 65-kDa hsp has 30% similarity at gapweight 10 with a human 70-kDa hsp. For immunologists it is particularly interesting to note that four regions made up of at least ten amino acid residues exist which are almost or fully identical (Table 1). It has been shown that immunogenic peptides of this length can bind directly to the MHC molecule without a requirement for endogenous processing (MacDonald and Nabholz 1986).

3.1 T-Cells from Normal Donors Recognize Self Epitopes of the 65-kDa hsp Shared by Man and Mycobacteria

On the basis of these observations the 65-kDa hsp appeared particularly suited for studying antigenic mimicry between microbial and host antigens and its possible relevance to autoimmune disease. As a first step along this line we wanted to address the question as to whether T cells with specificity to self epitopes of the 65-kDa hsp shared by microbes and the host exist in normal individuals (Munk et al. 1989). Peripheral blood monocytes from healthy donors were purified over Ficoll, and afterwards T-cell lines were established by stimulation with killed *M. tuberculosis*. These T-cell lines, after 7 days of culture, were tested in a cytotoxicity assay using autologous adherent cells as targets. Targets had been pulsed with killed *M. tuberculosis*, with purified intact r65-kDa hsp of *M. bovis*/*M. tuberculosis*, or with tryptic fragments of this molecule. The T-cell lines were capable of lysing target cells pulsed with *M. tuberculosis* or with tryptic fragments of the 65-kDa hsp but not targets pulsed with the intact molecule. These findings suggest that killed *M. tuberculosis* activates T cells with specificity for epitopes of the 65-kDa hsp which are not revealed through endogenous processing of this molecule.

Could the self epitopes shared by the mycobacterial and human 65-kDa hsp be among them? To analyze this question, targets were labeled with four synthetic peptides corresponding to self-epitopes of the human 65-kDa hsp. T cells from different individuals, after activation with killed *M. tuberculosis*, had indeed

Table 2. T cells from healthy individuals after activation with killed *M. tuberculosis* organisms, lyse targets primed with *M. tuberculosis* and with synthetic peptides corresponding to shared self epitopes of the 65-kDa hsp[a]. (From MUNK et al. 1989)

Donor	Target cell treatment	Percent specific lysis at effector:target ratio			
		90:1	30:1	15:1	5:1
1	*M. tuberculosis*	24	14	17	4
	Peptide 109–120[b]	39	15	0	0
	Peptide 430–441	32	8	6	4
	Nil	6	0	1	0
2	*M. tuberculosis*	67	26	19	7
	Peptide 269–289	58	26	0	0
	Peptide 298–307	33	12	10	0
	Nil	5	3	0	0

[a]T cells from healthy individuals were activated with killed *M. tuberculosis* organisms, and afterwards their cytolytic activity was assessed using autologous adherent cells as targets. Targets were primed with killed *M. tuberculosis* or with peptides corresponding to self epitopes of the 65-KDa hsp shared by man and mycobacteria. Specific lysis was calculated as described (KAUFMANN et al. 1986)

[b]Residue number corresponds to human amino acid sequence of the 65-kDa hsp

gained specificity for one or more of these self epitopes (Table 2). Because three of the four self peptides are enclosed by trypsin cleavage sites (peptide 109–120, peptide 269–289, and peptide 430–441), they should also be present in the tryptic digest of the 65-kDa hsp. In subsequent studies we obtained evidence that the cytotoxic T-lymphocyte (CTL) activity was class II restricted. These findings argue for the existence of self-reactive T cells in healthy individuals. It appears that these self-reactive epitopes are not generated by natural processing of the bacterial 65-kDa hsp. They seem, however, to be present in the preparation of killed *M. tuberculosis* organisms used here. We know that this preparation contains a significant fraction of low molecular weight components. Hence it is possible that peptides comprising the shared epitopes had been generated through bacterial autolysis, and that these peptides could directly bind to the MHC, thus by-passing natural processing. Once activated, these CTL can recognize host cells labeled with synthetic self peptides.

Recently, strong evidence for clonal deletion of T cells with specificity for self epitopes has been presented (MACDONALD et al. 1988; KAPPLER et al. 1988). Our findings that T cells with specificity to shared epitopes of the human and mycobacterial 65-kDa hsp exist but fail to recognize target cells primed with the intact bacterial 65-kDa hsp are not incompatible with this notion. Rather, they could best be explained by the assumption that these self-reactive T cells can exist because the shared epitopes are not generated in sufficient density by endogenous processing. Obviously, this then raises the question of whether T cells to these self epitopes can be activated during infection.

3.2 Murine T Cells Raised Against the Mycobacterial 65-kDa hsp Recognize Stressed Macrophages

The second set of experiments addresses the question as to whether CTL with specificity for self peptides of the 65-kDa hsp recognize stressed host cells, and hence whether they can induce autoimmune responses in the absence of microbial antigens (KOGA et al. 1989). Screening different monoclonal antibodies (MAB) to the mycobacterial 65-kDa hsp, we identified one MAB which also reacted with a similar though slightly larger molecule in murine bone marrow derived macrophages (BMMØ). This MAB, designated IA10, was kindly provided by Dr. J. DEBRUYN (THOLE et al. 1988). Figure 2 shows a Western blot of lysates of murine BMMØ stained with the IA10 MAB. Flow cytometry of BMMØ with this antibody revealed low or nondetectable expression of the homologous epitope by unstimulated cells. In contrast, interferon-γ (IFN-γ) stimulated macrophages expressed the epitope recognized by MAB IA10. Taken together, these findings show: (a) that a molecule slightly larger than the mycobacterial 65-kDa hsp can be detected in unstimulated BMMØ by a MAB made against the mycobacterial 65-kDa hsp, and (b) that surface expression of this cross-reactive epitope is up-regulated in BMMØ by IFN-γ. These findings show that antibodies against a bacterial hsp recognize stressed, though not resting macrophages and hence could cause autoimmune reactions.

T cells fail to see their antigen directly. Rather, they are specific for antigenic peptides which are presented in the context of self MHC molecules. Murine T cells against tryptic fragments of the mycobacterial 65-kDa hsp were used to approach the question of whether self epitopes were also processed and presented in the context of MHC molecules. It has been shown recently that CD8^{+} CTL can be activated in vitro by coculture with high peptide concentrations (CARBONE et al.

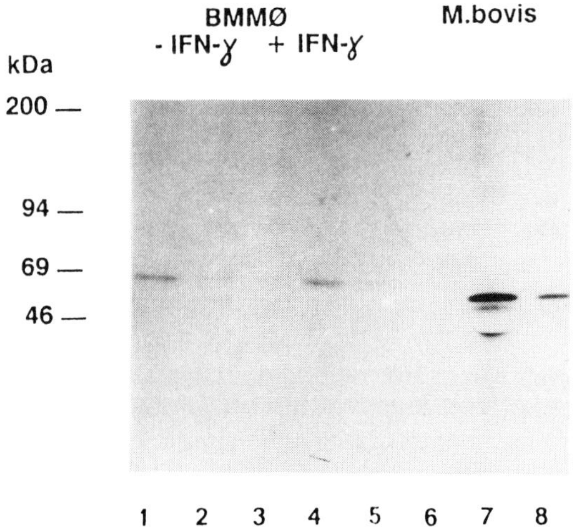

Fig. 2. Identification of a 65-kDa protein in murine BMMØ by staining with a MAB directed against the mycobacterial 65-kDa hsp. Descending concentrations of BMMØ lysate without (*1–3*) and with IFN-γ stimulation (*4–6*). *M. bovis* lysate as a positive control (*7, 8*)

Table 3. Murine T cells after activation with peptides of the mycobacterial 65-kDa hsp not only lyse BMMØ primed with these peptides but also stressed BMMØ in the absence of exogenous peptides[a]. (From KOGA et al. 1989)

BMMØ treatment	Percent specific lysis at effector:target ratio		
	60:1	20:1	7:1
Untreated	20	7	4
Priming with peptides of the 65-KDa hsp	62	39	28
Stress by IFN-γ	58	26	14

[a] T cells from normal mice were activated with tryptic fragments of the mycobacterial 65-kDa hsp, and afterwards their cytolytic activity was assessed in a ^{51}Cr-release assay. BMMØ after 9 days of in vitro culture in Teflon bags were left untreated, primed with a tryptic digest of the mycobacterial 65-kDa hsp, or stressed by IFN-γ-activation. Specific lysis was calculated as described (KAUFMANN et al. 1986)

1988). We applied this technique for activating T-cells with specificity to the 65-kDa hsp (KOGA et al. 1989). Murine spleen cells were cultured in the presence of a tryptic digest of the 65-kDa hsp of *M. bovis/M. tuberculosis.* After 6–8 days, the cytolytic activity of these T-cells was assessed using syngeneic BMMØ as targets which had been labeled with tryptic fragments of the mycobacterial 65-kDa hsp, stimulated with IFN-γ, or remained untreated. Not only BMMØ labeled with tryptic fragments of the 65-kDa hsp but also those activated by IFN-γ were recognized by the T-cell lines. In contrast, untreated BMMØ were not lysed (Table 3). Interestingly, BMMØ infected with cytomegalovirus were also recognized by CTL activated by the mycobacterial 65-kDa hsp (KOGA et al. 1989). The cytolytic activity observed here resided in the CD8$^+$ class I restricted T-cell set. CTL against the mycobacterial 65-kDa hsp failed to lyse BMMØ labeled with tryptic fragments of ovalbumin, and, conversely, CTL against ovalbumin failed to lyse BMMØ labeled with tryptic fragments of the 65-kDa hsp or IFN-γ activated BMMØ. We, therefore, believe that target cell recognition was antigen-specific. The most plausible explanation would be that IFN-γ activated BMMØ expressed a self epitope shared with mycobacteria in the context of the MHC class I molecule.

In this section we have shown: (a) that a cross-reactive B-cell epitope shared by the mycobacterial 65-kDa hsp and a host molecule of similar size is constitutively present in murine BMMØ; (b) that this epitope is expressed on the surface of stressed BMMØ; and (c) that a shared epitope, in the context of MHC class I molecules, is recognized by CTL directed against the 65-kDa hsp of mycobacteria. These data suggest that hsp may play a role in autoimmunity. Indeed, a role of the 65-kDa hsp in rheumatoid arthritis has been deduced from recent experimental and clinical studies (VAN EDEN et al. 1988; RES et al. 1988; HOLOSHITZ et al. 1989). Furthermore, autoantibodies to hsp are frequently found in systemic lupus erythematosus (MINOTA et al. 1988a, b).

3.3 *M. leprae* Primed and Stressed Schwann's Cells Are Lysed by T-lymphocytes

Schwann's cells are a major habitat of *M. leprae*, and Schwann's cell damage is a major pathogenic mechanism in leprosy (Kaufmann 1986; Ridley and Job 1985). Several lines of evidence indicate that Schwann's cell destruction is caused by immune mechanisms rather by than the pathogen itself (Ridley and Job 1985). One possible mechanism would be the destruction of Schwann's cells by CTL. To approach this question we established murine Schwann's cell cultures and assessed whether they could fulfill the prerequisite for interaction with CTL, i.e., whether they could phagocytose, process, and present mycobacterial antigens to CTL. Schwann's cells were infected with viable *M. leprae* (kindly provided by Dr. J. Kazda). Afterwards, cultures were stained by the Gomory reaction. Electron microscopy revealed that Schwann's cells were heavily infected with *M. leprae*. The microbes were found lying inside phagosomes which were surrounded by electron-dense material indicating acid phosphatase accumulation (Steinhoff et al. 1989; Fig. 3). This finding suggests fusion of lysosomes with phagosomes containing *M. leprae*.

Schwann's cells were stained with MAB against MHC class I or class II MAB. Schwann's cells lacked not only MHC class II but also MHC class I surface expression (Steinhoff and Kaufmann 1988). However, after IFN-γ stimulation Schwann's cells expressed a remarkable level of MHC class I molecules. Thus, at least after IFN-γ activation, murine Schwann's cells fulfilled the prerequisites for antigen-specific interaction with CD8 T-lymphocytes. Hence we pursued our strategy by asking whether CTL of CD8 phenotype would recognize and kill Schwann's cells presenting *M. leprae* antigens (kindly provided by Dr. P. Brennan). As shown in Table 4, Schwann's cells primed with *M. leprae* or stimulated with rIFN-γ were not killed, whereas IFN-γ stimulated and *M. leprae* primed Schwann's cells were effectively lysed (Steinhoff and Kaufmann 1988). These results are compatible with the idea that CTL can cause nerve damage. Nerve damage is a characteristic feature of both lepromatous and tuberculoid leprosy (Ridley and Job 1985). In tuberculoid leprosy strong T-cell responses and only few *M. leprae* organisms are observed; in particular, Schwann's cells are only rarely infected with *M. leprae*. Hence, in this situation, the antigen is rare or absent. How then could Schwann's cell lysis by CTL occur? Perhaps CTL directed against cross-reactive epitopes of hsp provide the missing link.

If this is the case, IFN-γ stimulation should induce increased surface expression of both the class I restriction element and the cross-reactive peptide. Indeed, CTL raised against tryptic fragments of the mycobacterial 65-kDa hsp lysed IFN-γ stimulated Schwann's cells in the absence of peptides of the 65-kDa hsp, and lysis was further elevated when these peptides were added (Table 5). In contrast, CTL raised against a tryptic digest of ovalbumin failed to kill IFN-γ stimulated Schwann's cells but did so after addition of tryptic ovalbumin peptides. Lytic activity was a function of $CD8^+$ T cells. Our studies in the murine Schwann's cell model, therefore, could provide an explanation for nerve destruction by *M. leprae* reactive CTL even of Schwann's cells which do not harbor *M. leprae* organisms.

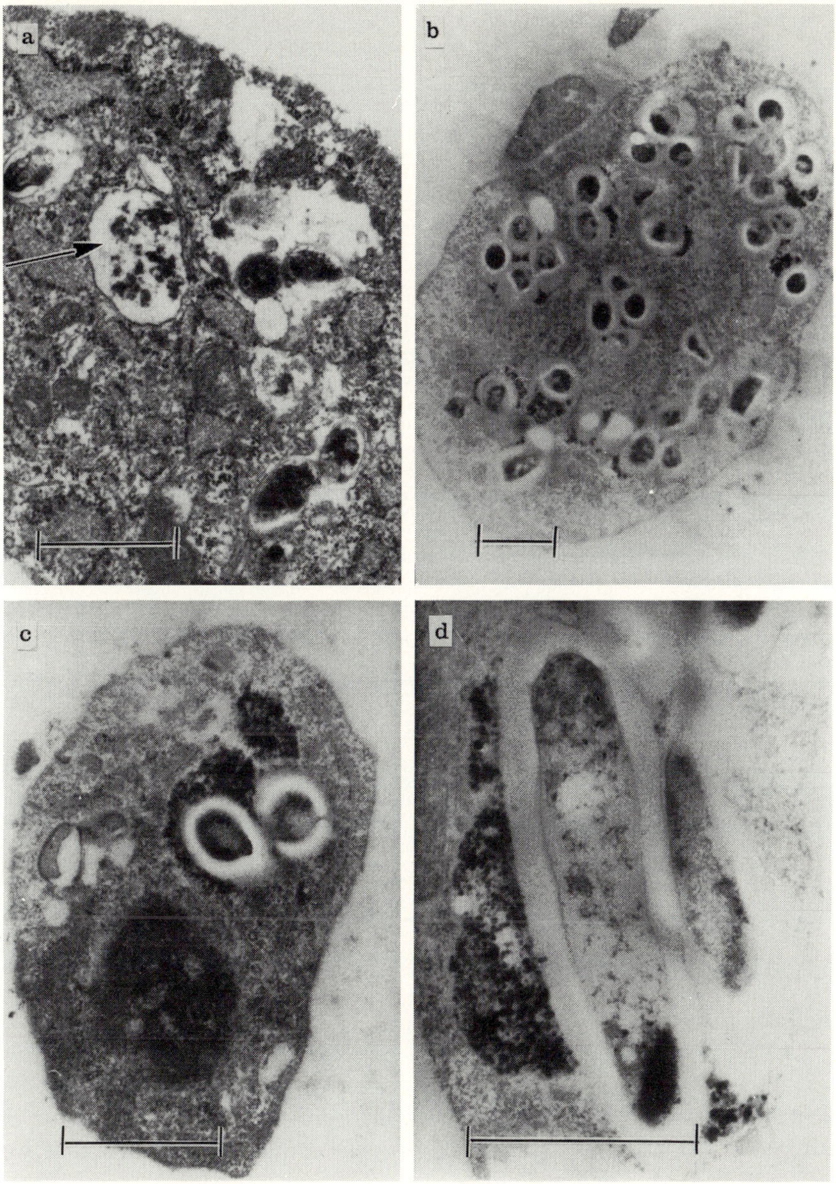

Fig. 3a–d. Evidence for phagosome-lysosome fusion in *M. leprae* infected Schwann's cells. Schwann's cells which were infected for 72 h with viable *M. leprae* organisms at a ratio of 20 bacteria to one Schwann's cell were stained for the lysosomal enzyme acid phosphatase. Accumulation of this enzyme next to the bacilli-containing phagosomes indicates phagosome-lysosome fusion. **a** Degraded material (*arrow*), perhaps originating from *M. leprae*, in the lysosome of a Schwann's cell not stained for acid phosphatase. **b** Deposits of acid phosphatase in close contact with the electron-transparent zone surrounding *M. leprae* organisms. **c, d** Multiple deposits of the lysosomal enzyme in heavily infected Schwann's cells. *Bars*, 1 μm. (From STEINHOFF et al. 1989, with permission)

Table 4. Murine T cells with reactivity to *M. leprae* lyse Schwann's cells stimulated with IFN-γ and primed with killed *M. leprae* organisms. (From STEINHOFF and KAUFMANN 1988)

Schwann's cell treatment	Percent specific lysis at effector:target ratio	
	20:1	10:1
Stimulation with IFN-γ	1	1
Priming with killed *M. leprae*	8	7
Stimulation with IFN-γ plus priming with the killed *M. leprae*	30	18

T cells from mice immunized with killed *M. leprae* were long-term cultured in the presence of syngeneic accessory cells, killed *M. leprae*, and crude T-cell growth factors. Schwann's cell cultures were established as described (STEINHOFF et al. 1989) and then were stimulated with IFN-γ alone, primed with killed *M. leprae*, or stimulated with IFN-γ and primed with *M. leprae*. Specific lysis was determined as described (KAUFMANN et al. 1986).

Table 5. Murine T cells after activation with peptides of the mycobacterial 65-kDa hsp not only lyse Schwann's cell primed with these peptides but also stressed Schwann's cells
Schwann's cell cultures were established as described (STEINHOFF and KAUFMANN 1988) and then were used as targets of T cells which had been activated with tryptic fragments of the 65-kDa hsp. Specific lysis was determined as described (KAUFMANN et al. 1986)

Schwann's cell treatment	Percent specific lysis at effector:target ratio	
	60:1	20:1
Untreated	23%	12%
Priming with peptides of the 65-kDA hsp plus IFN-γ	87%	61%
Stress by IFN-γ activation	77%	54%

4 Concluding Remarks

We have provided evidence here—though not full proof—to suggest a role of hsp in the pathogenesis of mycobacterial infections. The sequence of events that we envisage could be formulated as follows:

1. Mycobacteria stressed by host factors produce abundant hsp to protect themselves from host defence mechanisms.
2. Hsp are degraded into immunogenic peptides either (a) by the endogenous processing machinery of host cells or (b) by bacterial proteases through an autolytic pathway.
3. Immunogenic peptides include epitopes shared with host components.
4. These can be presented in the context of MHC molecules and hence autoreactive T cells can be activated.

5. Host cells stressed by a variety of insults produce their own hsp to protect themselves.
6. Shared epitopes derived from self hsp are processed and presented in the context of MHC molecules.
7. In this way, T cells which had been activated by shared epitopes derived from mycobacterial hsp can sense stressed host cells and interact with them.
8. This could initiate a sequence of auto-reactive events.

According to the data shown here, CD4 and CD8 T-lymphocytes might be involved. Very recent evidence indicates that, in addition to these conventional T cells expressing the α/β T-cell receptor, also T cells expressing the γ/δ T-cell receptor can recognize mycobacterial components and perhaps 65-kDa hsp (HOLOSHITZ et al. 1989; O'BRIEN et al. 1989; JANIS et al. 1989; MODLIN et al. 1989). These γ/δ T-cells may also contribute to autoimmune sequelae of mycobacterial infections.

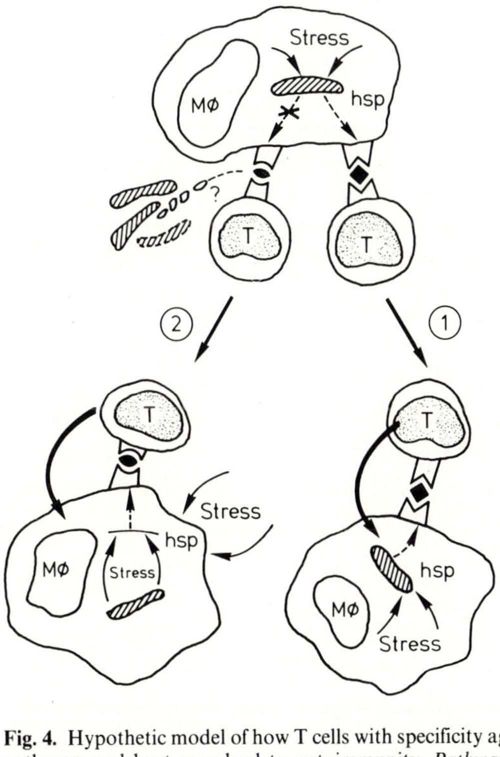

Fig. 4. Hypothetic model of how T cells with specificity against epitopes shared by the 65-kDa hsp from pathogen and host may lead to autoimmunity. *Pathway 1* illustrates the activation of T cells which recognize epitopes of bacterial hsp only. *Pathway 2* depicts the activation of T cells with specificity for a cross-reactive self epitope. Current evidence suggests that these self epitopes are not produced through natural processing. Rather, other ways of peptide generation must be assumed. One possibility would be the generation of peptides through autolytic degradation and the subsequent binding to the MHC molecule. Once activated by bacterial epitopes, such T cells could recognize stressed host cells presenting self epitope derived from endogenous hsp and shared with the bacterial hsp. *MΦ*, Macrophage; *hsp*, heat shock protein; *T*, T-cell

The previous finding from our laboratory that approximately 20% of murine T cells which respond to *M. tuberculosis* are specific for the mycobacterial 65-kDa hsp suggests that this molecule is an immunodominant T-cell antigen (KAUFMANN et al. 1987). Furthermore, our finding that peripheral blood T-lymphocytes from many healthy individuals recognize the mycobacterial 65-kDa hsp and even respond to shared epitopes of this antigen after appropriate stimulation in vitro suggests that this molecule is a common antigen, probably because it is present in many if not all microbes (MUNK et al. 1989; KAUFMANN 1989).

Why then is it that most individuals do not develop autoimmune disease although they may possess T cells of this self-specificity? Evidence has been presented that T cells with specificity for frequent and readily available self epitopes are deleted during their maturation (MACDONALD et al. 1988; KAPPLER et al. 1988). Since T cells directed against self epitopes of hsp can be readily demonstrated we must reject the notion that these peptides are generated in the high density required for T-cell deletion in the thymus or T-cell activation in the periphery. If these peptides would only derive from self molecules, the host would be safe. The high conservation of hsp, however, provides for another source of self epitopes, namely shared epitopes of bacterial origin. For these epitopes to be immunogenic they must be generated in sufficient amounts and then bound to the MHC molecule. Our data suggest that self epitopes of the 65-kDa hsp are processed and presented in the context of MHC molecules in a density which is sufficient for T-cell recognition. Activation of T cells may, however, require a higher epitope density which is not readily achieved through natural processing. Perhaps shared self epitopes are derived from bacterial hsp which are degraded through an autolytic process at sites suffering from a high bacterial load. Provided that at certain stages of infection shared peptides are generated, this incident could evoke a sequence of events which ultimately leads to autoimmunity (see Fig. 4).

Acknowledgements. The valuable help of Drs. J.D.A. van Embden, J. DeBruyn, J. Kazda, P. Brennan, S. Modrow, and R.A. Young is gratefully acknowledged. rIFN-γ was produced by Genentech and kindly provided by Boehringer Ingelheim. Appreciation is also extended to U. Väth, C. Kronfeld, D. Preuss, and R. Mahmoudi.

References

Bardwell JCA, Craig EA (1984) Major heat-shock gene of *Drosophila* and *Escherichia coli* heat-inducible *dnaK* gene are homologous. Proc Natl Acad Sci USA 81: 848–852

Bardwell JCA, Craig EA (1987) Eukaryotic M_r 83,000 heat shock protein has a homologue in *Escherichia coli*. Proc Natl Acad Sci USA 84: 5177–5181

Carbone FR, Moore MW, Sheil JM, Bevan MJ (1988) Induction of cytotoxic T lymphocytes by primary in vitro stimulation with peptides. J Exp Med 167: 1767–1779

Chirico WJ, Waters MG, Blobel G (1988) 70K heat shock related proteins stimulate protein translocation into microsomes. Nature 332: 805–810

Christman MF, Morgan RW, Jacobson FS, Ames BN (1985) Positive control of a regulon for defenses against oxidative stress and some heat-shock proteins in *Salmonella typhimurium*. Cell 41: 753–762

Collins PL, Hightower LE (1982) Newcastle disease virus stimulates the cellular accumulation of stress (heat shock) mRNAs and proteins. J Virol 44: 703–707

Craig EA (1985) The heat shock response. CRC Crit Rev Biochem 18: 239–280

Deshaies RJ, Koch BD, Werner-Washburne M, Craig EA, Schekman R (1988) A subfamily of stress proteins facilitates translocation of secretory and mitochondrial precursor polypeptides. Nature 332: 800–805

Ellis J (1987) Proteins as molecular chaperones. Nature 328: 378–379

Emmrich F, Thole J, van Embden J, Kaufmann SHE (1986) A recombinant 64 kilo Dalton protein of *Mycobacterium bovis* BCG specifically stimulated human T4 clones reactive to mycobacterial antigens. J Exp Med 163: 1024–1029

Ferris DK, Harel-Bellan A, Morimoto RI, Welch WJ, Farrar WL (1988) Mitogen and lymphokine stimulation of heat shock proteins in T lymphocytes. Proc Natl Acad Sci USA 85: 3850–3854

Fields PI, Swanson RV, Haidaris CG, Heffrow F (1986) Mutants of *Salmonella typhimurium* that cannot survive within the macrophage are avirulent. Proc Natl Acad Sci USA 83: 5189–5193

Garry RF, Ulug ET, Bose HR (1983) Induction of stress proteins in Sindbis virus- and vesicular stomatitis virus-infected cells. Virology 129: 319–332

Garsia RJ, Hellqvist L, Booth RJ, Radford AJ, Britton WJ, Astbury L, Trent RJ, Basten A (1989) Homology of the 70-kilodalton antigens from *Mycobacterium leprae* and *Mycobacterium bovis* with the *Mycobacterium tuberculosis* 71-kilodalton antigen and with the conserved heat shock protein 70 of eukaryotes. Infect Immun 57: 204–212

Gerner EW, Boone R, Connor WG, Hicks JA, Boone MLM (1976) A transient thermotolerant survival response produced by single thermal doses in HeLa cells. Cancer Res. 36: 1035–1040

Hahn H, Kaufmann SHE (1981) Role of cell-mediated immunity in bacterial infections. Rev Infect Dis 3: 1221–1250

Hansen K, Bangsborg JM, Fjordvang H, Strandberg-Pedersen N, Hindersson P (1988) Immunochemical characterization of and isolation of the gene for a *Borrelia burgdorferi* immunodominant 60-kilodalton antigen common to a wide range of bacteria. Infect Immun 56: 2047–2053

Hemmingsen SM, Woolford C, van der Vies SM, Tilly K, Dennis DT, Georgopoulos CP, Hendrix RW, Ellis RJ (1988) Homologous plant and bacterial proteins chaperone oligomeric protein assembly. Nature 333: 330–334

Henle KJ, Leeper DB (1976) Interaction of hyperthermia and radiation in CHO cells: recovery kinetics. Radiat Res 66: 505–518

Hindersson P, Knudsen JD, Axelsen NH (1987) Cloning and expression of *Treponema pallidum* common antigen (Tp-4) in *E. coli* K-12. J Gen Microbiol 133: 587–596

Holoshitz J, Koning F, Coligan JE, DeBruyn J, Strober S (1989) Isolation of $CD4^-$ $CD8^-$ mycobacteria-reactive T lymphocyte clones from rheumatoid arthritis synovial fluid. Nature 339: 226–229

Janis E, Kaufmann SHE, Schwartz RH, Pardoll DM (1989) Activation of $\gamma\delta^+$ T cells in the primary immune response to *Mycobacterium tuberculosis*. Science 244: 713–716

Jindal S, Dudani AK, Harley CB, Singh B, Gupta RS (1989) Primary structure of a human mitochondrial protein homologous to the bacterial and plant chaperonins and to the 65-kilodalton mycobacterial antigen. Mol Cell Biol 9: 2279–2283

Kappler JW, Staerz U, White J, Marrack P (1988) Self-tolerance eliminates T cells specific for Mls-modified products of the major histocompatibility complex. Nature 332: 35–40

Kaufmann SHE (1986) Immunology of leprosy: new facts, future perspectives. Microb Pathogen 1: 107–114

Kaufmann SHE (1987) Towards new leprosy and tuberculosis vaccines. Microbiol Sci 4: 324–328

Kaufmann SHE (1989) Immunity to bacteria and fungi. Curr Opin Immunol 1: 431–440

Kaufmann SHE, Hug E, DeLibero G (1986) *Listeria monocytogenes* reactive T lymphocyte clones with cytolytic activity against infected target cells. J Exp Med 164: 363–368

Kaufmann SHE, Väth U, Thole JER, van Embden JDA, Emmrich F (1987) Ennumeration of T cells reactive with *Mycobacterium tuberculosis* organisms and specific for the recombinant mycobacterial 64 kiloDalton protein. Eur J Immunol 17: 351–357

Khandjian EW, Türler H (1983) Simian virus 40 and polyoma virus induce synthesis of heat shock proteins in permissive cells. Mol Cell Biol 3: 1–8

Koga T, Wand-Württenberger A, DeBruyn J, Munk ME, Schoel B, Kaufmann SHE (1989) T cells and antibodies against a common bacterial heat shock protein recognize stressed macrophages. Science 245: 1112–1115

Lamb JR, Ivanyi J, Rees ADM, Rothbard JB, Howland K, Young RA, Young DB (1987) Mapping of T cell epitopes using recombinant antigens and synthetic peptides. EMBO J 6: 1245–1249

LaThangue NB, Latchman DS (1987) Nuclear accumulation of a heat-shock 70-like protein during herpes simplex virus replication. Biosci 7: 475–483

LaThangue NB, Shriver K, Dawson C, Chan WL (1984) Herpes simplex virus infection causes the accumulation of a heat-shock protein. EMBO J 3: 267–277

Lindquist S (1986) The heat shock response. Annu Rev Biochem 55: 1151–1191

MacDonald HR, Nabholz M (1986) T-cell activation, Annu Rev Cell Biol 2: 231–253

MacDonald HR, Schneider R, Lees R, Howe RC, Achaorbea H, Festenstein H, Zinkernagel RM, Hengartner H (1988) T-cell receptor V-beta use predicts reactivity and tolerance to Mls-alpha-encoded antigens. Nature 332: 40–45

McMullin TW, Hallberg RL (1988) A highly evolutionarily conserved mitochondrial protein is structurally related to the protein encoded by the *E. coli groEL* gene. Mol Cell Biol 8: 371–380

Minota S, Cameron B, Welch WJ, Winfield JB (1988a) Autoantibodies to the constitutive 73-kD member of the hsp70 family of heat shock proteins in systemic lupus erythematosus. J Exp Med 168: 1475–1480

Minota S, Koyasu S, Yahara I, Winfield J (1988b) Autoantibodies to the heat-shock protein hsp 90 in systemic lupus erythematosus. J Clin Invest 81: 106–109

Modlin RL, Pirmez C, Hofman FM, Torigian V, Uyemura K, Rea TH, Bloom BR, Brenner MB (1989) Antigen-specific T cell receptor $\gamma\delta$ bearing lymphocytes accumulate in human infectious disease lesions. Nature 339: 544–548

Modrow S, Höflacher B, Mellert W, Erfle V, Wahren B, Wolf H (1989) Use of synthetic oligopeptides in identification and characterization of immunological functions in the amino acid sequence of the envelope protein of HIV-1. J Acquired Imm Def Syndr 2: 120–127

Morgan RW, Christman MF, Jacobson FS, Storz G, Ames BN (1986) Hydrogen peroxide-inducible proteins in *Salmonella typhimurium* overlap with heat shock and other stress proteins. Proc Natl Acad Sci USA 83: 8059–8063

Moulder JW (1985) Comparative biology of intracellular parasitism. Microbiol Rev 49: 298–337

Munk ME, Schoel B, Kaufmann SHE (1988) T cell responses of normal individuals towards recombinant protein antigens of *Mycobacterium tuberculosis*. Eur J Immunol 18: 1835–1838

Munk ME, Schoel B, Modrow S, Karr RW, Young RA, Kaufmann SHE (1989) Cytolytic $CD4^+$ T lymphocytes from healthy individuals with specificity to self epitopes shared by the mycobacterial and human 65 kDa heat shock protein. J Immunol (in press)

Nevins JR (1982) Induction of the synthesis of a 70,000 dalton mammalian heat shock protein by the adenovirus E1A gene product. Cell 29: 913–919

Newport GR, Culpepper J, Agabian N (1988) Heat shock response and parasitism. Parasitol Today 4: 306–312

Notarianni EL, Preston CM (1982) Activation of cellular stress protein genes by herpes simplex virus temperature-sensitive mutants which overproduce immediate early polypeptides. Virology 123: 113–122

O'Brien RL, Happ MP, Dallas A, Palmer E, Kubo R, Born WK (1989) Stimulation of a major subset of lymphocytes expressing T cell receptor $\gamma\delta$ by an antigen-derived *Mycobacterium tuberculosis*. Cell 57: 667–674

Oftung F, Mustafa AS, Husson R, Young RA, Godal T (1987) Human T cell clones recognize two abundant *Mycobacterium tuberculosis* protein antigens expressed in *Escherichia coli*. J Immunol 138: 927–931

Ottenhoff THM, Kale Ab B, van Embden JDA, Thole JER, Kiessling R (1988) The recombinant 65 kilodalton heat shock protein of *Mycobacterium bovis* BCG/*M. tuberculosis* is a target molecule for $CD4^+$ cytotoxic T lymphocytes that lyse human monocytes. J Exp Med 168: 1947

Pelham H (1988) Coming in from the cold. Nature 332: 776–777

Polla BS (1988) A role for heat shock proteins in inflammation? Immunol Today 9: 134–137

Polla BS, Healy AM, Wojno WC, Krane SM (1987) Hormone 1α, 25-di-hydroxyvitamin D_3 modulated heat shock response in monocytes. Am J Physical 252: C640–C649

Res PCM, Schaar CG, Breedveld FC, van Eden W, van Embden JDA, Cohen IR, de Vries RRP (1988) Synovial fluid T cell reactivity against 65 kD heat shock protein of mycobacteria in early chronic arthritis. Lancet ii: 478–480

Ridley DS, Job CK (1985) The pathology of leprosy. In: Hastings RC (ed) Leprosy. Churchill Livingstone, Edinburgh

Shinnick TM (1987) The 65-kilodalton antigen of *Mycobacterium tuberculosis*. J Bacteriol 169: 1080–1088

Shinnick TM, Vodkin MH, Williams JL (1988) The *Mycobacterium tuberculosis* 65 kDa antigen is a heat shock protein which corresponds to common antigen and to the *E. coli* groEL protein. Infect Immun 56: 446–451

Steinhoff U, Kaufmann SHE (1988) Specific lysis by $CD8^+$ T cells of Schwann cells expressing *Mycobacterium leprae* antigens. Eur J Immunol 18: 973–976

Steinhoff U, Golecki JR, Kazda J, Kaufmann SHE (1989) Evidence for phagosome lysosome fusion in *Mycobacterium leprae* infected murine Schwann cells. Infect Immun 57: 1008–1010

Thole JER, KeulenWJ, Kolk AHJ, Groothuis DG, Berwald LG, Tiesjema RH, van Embden JDA (1987) Characterization, sequence determination, and immunogenicity of a 64-kilodalton protein of *Mycobacterium bovis* BCG expressed in *Escherichia coli* K-12. Infect Immun 55: 1466–1475

Thole JER, Hindersson P, DeBruyn J, Cremers F, van der Zee J, de Cock H, Tommassen J, van Eden W, van Embden JDA (1988) Antigenic relatedness of a strongly immunogenic 65 kDa mycobacterial protein antigen with a similarly sized ubiquitous bacterial common antigen. Microb Pathogen 4: 71–83

Ungewickell E (1985) The 70 kDa mammalian heat shock proteins are structurally and functionally related to the uncoating protein that releases clathrin triskelia from coated vesicles. EMBO J 4: 3385–3391

Van Buskirk A, Crump BL, Pierce SK (1989) A peptide binding protein having a role in antigen presentation is a member of the hsp 70 heat shock family. J Exp Med (in press)

Van Eden W, Thole JER, van der Zee R, Noordzij A, van Embden JDA, Hensen EJ, Cohen IR (1988) Cloning of the mycobacterial epitope recognized by T lymphocytes in adjuvant arthritis. Nature 331: 171–173

Vodkin MH, Williams JC (1988) A heat shock operon in *Coxiella burnetii* produces a major antigen homologous to a protein in both mycobacteria and *Escherichia coli*. J Bacteriol 170: 1227–1234

Young DB, Ivanyi J, Cox JH, Lamb JR (1987) Th 65 kDa antigen of mycobacteria—a common bacterial protein? Immunol Today 8: 215–219

Young D, Lathigra R, Hendrix R, Sweetser D, Young RA (1988) Stress proteins are immune targets in leprosy and tuberculosis. Proc Natl Acad Sci USA 85: 4267–4270

Prediction and Identification of Bacterial and Parasitic T-Cell Antigens and Determinants

J. B. ROTHBARD[1] and J. R. LAMB[2]

1 Introduction

T-lymphocytes are integral in the generation of virtually all the effector functions of the vertebrate immune response. They can be divided broadly into two populations based on the surface expression of either the CD4 or CD8 glycoprotein (LITTMAN 1987). Even though both groups can be subdivided further based on the differential expression of other cell surface proteins and their ability to secrete different lymphokines (MOSSMAN and COFFMAN 1987), the CD4-positive cells are a useful demarcation because they regulate a variety of different cell types. They secrete a variety of T-cell growth factors, principally interleukin 2 (IL-2), which are required for the expansion of both CD4 and CD8 cells. In addition, they support the induction of immunoglobulin synthesis by B cells (HOWARD and PAUL 1983) and influence macrophage activation (UNANUE 1984). Consequently in order logically to modulate the immune response of an individual, the proteins and the particular determinants involved in the generation of the T-cell response must be defined. Even though protective immunity can be generated without this understanding it is required both to improve the efficacy and to reduce harmful side effects of vaccination.

2 Molecular Basis of T-Cell Antigen Recognition

In the past 3 years a unified model of T-cell recognition of protein antigens has been developed based on the contributions of several laboratories (MOLLER 1987). In contrast with antibodies, and consequently B cells, T-lymphocytes are not stimulated by proteins in their native conformation. Instead, the antigen-specific receptor of T cells recognises linear fragments of protein immunogens in a complex with either MHC class I or II molecules. A significant advance in our understanding of the ternary complex formed between the T-cell receptor, peptide, and the MHC

[1] Molecular Immunology Laboratory, Imperial Cancer Research Fund, Lincoln's Inn Fields, London WC2A 3PX, UK

[2] MRC External Scientific Staff, Department of Immunology, Royal Postgraduate Medical School, Hammersmith Hospital, DuCane Road, London W12 OHS, UK

Current Topics in Microbiology and Immunology, Vol. 155

protein was the solution of the crystal structure of HLA-A2 (Bjorkman et al. 1987a, b). Not only did this provide the three-dimensional structure of a member of this highly homologous family, on which other alleles could be modelled, but it also provided evidence identifying a potential antigen combining site. In the X-ray diffraction map of the crystal, electron density approximately as great as in the rest of the structure but not covalently connected with the molecule was found in a central groove formed by two helical regions on top of an eight-standard β-pleated sheet. This observation coupled with the presence of the vast majority of the polymorphic residues in the molecule either within or lining the site has led to the conclusion not only that peptide is bound in this region, but also that this site is occupied with endogenous peptides in the majority of MHC molecules.

Direct binding of immunogenic peptides to purified, detergent-solubilised MHC class II molecules has been demonstrated using equilibrium dialysis (Babbitt et al. 1985) and gel filtration (Buus et al. 1986). Perhaps one of the most interesting features of these experiments was the observed kinetics of binding. Extremely slow rates of association and dissociation were found. This was not simply a function of using detergent-solubilised molecules because similar rates were found when the class II molecules were either immobilized in a lipid monolayer or expressed on cell surfaces (Watts et al. 1985; Busch et al. 1989).

The kinetics were not the only feature that distinguished the MHC molecules from other known receptors. The other unusual feature was their capacity to bind a wide diversity of peptides (Buus et al. 1987; Busch et al. 1989). The molecular basis of this degeneracy is not completely understood, however we have speculated that the many peptides might bind with a similar conformation and perhaps in a preferred location in the proposed antigen combining site (Rothbard and Taylor 1988). This premise was based on the presence of structural similarities found in the primary structure of a high percentage of the defined T-cell determinants (Rothbard and Taylor 1988; Spouge et al. 1987). These empirical observations have been partially confirmed by identifying residues critical for T-cell recognition by exchanging amino acids between two peptides capable of binding a common MHC protein (Rothbard et al. 1988, 1989). In addition, the development of an assay to detect MHC-peptide complexes on cell surfaces has revealed that many peptides can bind all 22 DR types examined.

As discussed in greater detail below, these theories have led to molecular models of the MHC-peptide complex, from which potentially important MHC residues in binding can be identified. If these models are generalizable, they should greatly improve the ability to identify peptides that can bind MHC proteins with high affinity in the primary sequence of any protein.

3 T-Cell Recognition of Microbial Antigens

While the experiments discussed above have provided considerable information on the physical nature of peptide-MHC interactions, they do not address the issue of how and where in the cell the complex is formed (Germain 1986). In addition, even though peptides from the same protein have been shown to compete for binding to MHC class II proteins (GAMMON et al. 1987; ADORINI et al. 1988), demonstrating affinity for MHC is a factor in deciding which part of a protein will be immunodominant, we still have a poor understanding of the factors involved in determining which protein of a complicated bacteria or parasite will be most important in the immune response.

In the past, defining determinants was necessary to generalize about T-cell recognition and understand the details of MHC-peptide complex (DELISI and BERZOFSKY 1985; ROTHBARD and TAYLOR 1988). However, at the present time identifying the most immunodominant proteins is far more important than simply collecting T-cell determinants in a particular system.

What are the factors that dictate which fragments of which proteins occupy the MHC combining site and consequently are dominant in the cellular immune response against a pathogen? Are there groups of proteins that predominate the responses to many bacteria and parasites? If so, can they be predicted a priori? Or will responsiveness and the details of the infection differ sufficiently between individuals that such generalizations will not be possible?

Currently these questions cannot be answered, however investigation of the T-cell response to mycobacteria has led to a number of interesting observations. The strategy developed by several laboratories was to identify the proteins recognized by antibodies from the serum of infected individuals (IVANYI et al. 1988). These proteins were then assumed also to be the principal stimulators of the $CD4^+$ T-cell population. Dissection of these molecules using deletion mutants and synthetic peptides has led to the identification of variety of linear T-cell determinants (MUSTAFA et al. 1986; OTTENHOFF et al. 1986; LAMB et al. 1986). These in turn were tested for their ability to stimulate human peripheral blood lymphocytes from several individuals and were shown to be commonly recognized. Subsequent cloning and sequencing of these proteins revealed that they were members of a family of proteins whose expression was induced by chemical or physical stress of the cells (R.A. YOUNG et al. 1985a), b; D.B. YOUNG et al. 1988). A possible explanation for their immunodominance is that they have been shown to function in intracellular transport and thus may be present at disproportionally high concentrations in the lysosome or other cell organelles where the peptide-MHC complex is formed. Whether this will be true of all gram-negative bacteria or limited to mycobacteria remains to be established. However these results support the contention that such groups of immunodominant proteins do exist.

4 Experimental Strategies for the Identification of Immunologically Important Proteins Within a Pathogen

Both the strategy adopted and the ease of identification of the critical proteins depends on the facility with which the pathogen can be propagated. In those cases in which the bacteria or the parasite is readily available, such as *Escherichia coli* and *Salmonella*, serum from human or animal models can simply be screened on the components of the microorganism separated by a variety of biochemical techniques. A large number of individuals must be screened before a particular protein can be classified as immunodominant. An additional caveat is that even if an individual protein predominates a response, it might not be relevant for consideration in a potential vaccine because the size of the response might simply reflect an important mechanism of deception that the organism has evolved. Because linear fragments of proteins complexed by MHC molecules stimulate T-cell responses, the native conformation of the protein need not be preserved in their isolation (SHIMONKEVITZ et al. 1983). Consequently, methods using denaturing conditions such as sodium dodecylsulphate polyacrylamide gel electrophoresis (SDS-PAGE), that are very effective in separating proteins of similar molecular weight but result in irreversible denaturation of most structures, are ideal for studying T-cell responses.

4.1 Use of Nitrocellulose-Bound Antigen in T-Cell Proliferation Assays

Electrophoretic separation of complex mixtures of proteins and subsequent transfer to nitrocellulose has been used to circumvent the need to purify each component and has allowed the specificity of the T-cell repertoire to be investigated (LAMB et al. 1988a). Comparison of the patterns of proliferation of T cells isolated from different individuals has identified not only the predominant stimulatory proteins in both viral and bacterial systems but has also revealed the importance of the response on the level of the population. Similarly, by screening the mixture of proteins from two different strains of microorganism, common or strain-specific determinants can be identified. In addition, fractions that fail to stimulate proliferation can be examined for inhibitory effects. As useful as this technique is, technical problems such as the difficulty of transferring sufficient quantities of antigen to the solid support can result in the failure to identify relevant proteins. The recent introduction of an apparatus separating proteins electrophoretically and directly transferring them to microfuge tubes without SDS might make the technique more sensitive and also remove many of the current limitations (Applied Biosystems, Foster City, CA).

4.2 Recombinant DNA Antigens and Synthetic Peptides

For those cases in which the pathogen cannot be easily grown, alternative strategies for isolating the proteins must be employed. A good example of this is *Mycobacterium leprae*, where a DNA expression library had to be constructed because of difficulty in culturing the organism. Placing bacterial fragments of DNA into the appropriate expression vectors enabled both the human and murine immune responses to be probed. Such a strategy, although laborious, could be applicable to most microorganisms.

Recombinant DNA antigens, expressed either as fusion proteins or secreted as full-length sequences, can be recognized by T cells, and in some cases antibodies. Consequently they have been useful in the analysis of the immune response to a number of pathogens including mycobacteria (MUSTAFA et al. 1986; MEHRA et al.

1986; LAMB et al. 1986). The cloning of genomic DNA fragments of the major protein antigens of *M. leprae* and *M. tuberculosis* helped resolve the problem of limited availability of purified antigens for probing T-cell responses (R.A. YOUNG et al. 1985a, b). Furthermore, by constructing a DNA sublibrary T-cell determinants within a protein antigen can be mapped, as was demonstrated for the 65-kDa gene of *M. leprae* (LAMB et al. 1986). Adding cellular lysates of bacteria expressing these fragments of DNA to cultures of polyclonal and monoclonal T-cell populations has resulted in the identification of two regions of the 65-kDa protein containing T-cell determinants, 54–99 and 361–523. The importance of these regions was confirmed using synthetic peptides (LAMB et al. 1986). The T-cell determinant within the sequence 54–99 recognized by the individual investigated was mapped to residues 65–85, whereas that in the other fragment corresponded to amino acids 365–379. The detection of antigen expressed by recombinant gene libraries depends upon recognition by murine monoclonal antibodies, and because the T- and B-cell repertoires do not necessarily overlap, preselection with antibodies may bias the antigens available for screening the T-cell repertoire. Therefore, a more direct approach for selecting recombinant clones from a library is necessary to explore fully the T-cell repertoire, which the electrophoretic separation might provide.

4.3 Infected Cells As Targets of Cytotoxic T-Cell Recognition

Alternatively, naturally occurring infected cells can be used as reagents to propagate or screen lymphocytes for responsiveness. This is particularly important for $CD8^+$ cells (TOWNSEND and MCMICHAEL 1985) and has been shown most clearly using viral systems in which this population of cells has needed to be expanded prior to their ability to be assayed. Similarly, there are examples in which cells infected with microbial antigens can be recognized by specific $CD8^+$ T cells (KAUFMANN 1988). T cells from mice primed with mycobacteria lyse only bone marrow cells infected with the specific microbe. In addition, Schwann's cells, which provide a major habitat for *M. leprae* appear to be lysed by MHC class I restriced $CD8^+$ T cells.

Individual open reading frames of many viral proteins have been expressed in histocompatible cells by transfection or infection with vaccinia or other viral vectors and used as targets in T-cell cytotoxicity assays (TOWNSEND et al. 1988). However the selection of which proteins are potential targets is more complicated in the case of a bacterium with a large genome or a multicellular parasite.

4.4 Prediction of T-Cell Determinants in Proteins

At the present time, two methods are utilized to predict previously unidentified T-cell determinants. Both were based on empirical analysis of a limited number of sequences and were intimately linked with the practical desire to limit the expense and effort necessary for the identification of epitopes. Consequently, neither group responsible for the two methods has argued that their approach is optimal. Rather they have emphasized that each has led to practical successes and might be useful for many systems. In addition, both hope to identify possible important general features of peptide-MHC interactions.

The emphasis in the respective algorithms is quite different—even though, in the end, their ideas have identified many common areas of proteins. DeLisi and Berzofsky (1985) initially postulated that many of the determinants defined at the time of their analysis could be folded into a helical structure, with the hydrophobic residues segregated from the hydrophilic amino acids. Believing such amphipathic character to be integral in T-cell recognition, by allowing the peptide selectively to interact either with the membrane or the MHC protein they developed a programme which identified regions in protein sequences displaying this characteristic. As previously mentioned, they have used the algorithm to identify T-cell determinants in several systems, including the circumsporozoite protein of malaria and the envelope protein of HTLV (Good et al. 1987; Cease et al. 1987).

In contrast, the approach taken by Rothbard and Taylor (1988) initially did not consider the secondary structure of the bound peptide. They reasoned that if the vast majority of determinants corresponded to linear sequences from the intact proteins, and the formation of a peptide-MHC complex was a necessary requirement for immune responsiveness, then characteristic patterns of amino acids should be present in the primary sequence of the determinants. Within this assumption, there are at least two other additional assumptions: (a) the ease of identification will be closely linked to the diversity both in the number of different conformations the peptides can bind and the number of possible locations that are present in the antigen combining site of the MHC proteins; and (b) each peptide must share structural similarity, but not necessarily identity, to allow it to bind the MHC molecules.

Initial observations identified two adjacent hydrophobic residues by which each of the approximately 30 helper and cytotoxic T-cell determinants could be aligned. In each case, these two residues were preceded by either a charged residue or a glycine. The pattern of three amino acids occurred sufficiently often in protein sequences that it had limited predictive value. To identify a rarer motif the fourth residue was considered. In approximately 75% of cases the next residue was polar. In the 25% where it was hydrophobic, in each case the next, or fifth, amino acid of the pattern was polar. These patterns of four or five linear amino acids coupled with the amino acid preferences at each position were incorporated into a program which not only identified them in a protein sequence but also ordered them based on their similarity to previously defined T-cell determinants. Such logic was integral in the identification of a relatively large number of both helper and cytotoxic determinants.

As the list of defined determinants increased, they could be segregated by restriction element and separately analysed. Again, aligning the sequences based on two adjacent hydrophobic residues, structural similarities were seen in a remarkably high number of determinants at positions flanking the hydrophobic amino acids. The similar residues were spaced at relative positions, 1, 4, 5 and 8, with the two hydrophobic amino acids imposing the central adjacent positions. Because these positions are juxtaposed when the peptide is folded into a helical conformation, this observation converges with the previously postulated association of T-cell determinants with a helical conformation.

As previously mentioned, the value of the proposed patterns was that they may allow us to identify an avenue for experimental investigation of the peptide-MHC complex. If valid, their presence suggests that there might be a preferred location and conformation for many peptides in the binding site. To test their utility, they were used to align peptide determinants recognized in the context of a common class II or class I protein. Based on the assumption that the structural similarities were critical for binding the restriction element, the dissimilar residues were exchanged between determinants to create hybrid peptides that in each case was shown to stimulate the appropriate T-cell clone. Consequently the strategy identified the minimum number of residues necessary for clonal specific recognition. In addition, the spacing of these residues placed restraints on the possible conformations which the bound peptide could adopt. Without a method initially to align the peptides, the number of ways in which amino acids composing the two peptides could be exchanged is so large as to be experimentally prohibitive. For example, two peptides composed of 12 amino acids aligned colinearly can generate 2^{12} (1096) different possible combinations of residues. If different alignments are considered even more possibilities exist.

As useful as these approaches were shown to be, several examples of peptides not exhibiting these general characteristics were known. In addition, several detailed investigations of individual determinants provided data arguing against a simple helical model for recognition.

An important advance in the understanding of peptide-MHC interactions has been related to the development of an assay for detecting peptide-MHC complexes on the surface of cells. Biotinylated peptides were incubated with B-cells lines expressing high levels of MHC class II proteins, washed, subsequently treated with flourescently labelled avidin, and assayed using flow cytometry (BUSCH et al. 1989). By placing the relatively large lysyl-biotin at each position in the peptide, distinct differences in binding were apparent that have been difficult to obtain with substitutions of any of the naturally occurring amino acids. The variations in observed flourescence were shown to be due to the modification with lysyl-biotin specifically affecting the peptide's affinity for the MHC protein. Biotinylation was shown not to affect detectably the conformation of the peptide, nor its susceptibility to proteases—two other reasonable explanations for the experimentally observed differences in binding. Consequently, this simple assay provided a quantitative measure of the importance of each amino acid in the formation of the complex. The size the flourescent signal was inversely related to importance of the residue in the interaction.

In the initial case examined the pattern of fluorescence was consistent, with the central nine residues of the determinant adopting a helical conformation and with the amino acids composing both the amino and carboxyl termini exhibiting greater conformational freedom. Examination of the ability of analogues containing point substitutions to either bind or be recognized by the T-cell receptor of an individual clone has provided information of the chemical and physical requirements of each position in the peptide. Taken together, this data has allowed a tentative model of the peptide in the binding site to be constructed. In the model, the three most critical residues interact with amino acids which exhibit differences in polymorphism. Two are proposed to interact with very polymorphic amino acids in the β-chain helix, residues 67 and 71, whereas the third is believed to interact with a conserved negative charge at position 15 in the α-chain (ROTHBARD et al. 1989). If valid, motifs can easily be constructed to reflect the hierarchy of interactions that will lead to high-affinity interactions, which in turn, should lead to extremely accurate predictions of peptides that can bind well.

5 Concluding Comments

The past few years have seen a dramatic advance in our understanding of T-cell recognition of protein antigens (MOLLER 1987; BJORKMAN et al. 1987a, b). Consequently, with this information experimental approaches for the modulation of immune responses can be logically designed. Technical advances in the electrophoretic separation of antigenic components and assays for determining the binding of peptides to MHC class II proteins expressed on the surface of cells allow the response to bacteria and parasites to be dissected and the critical proteins and fragments to be identified. Nevertheless, to use this information to generate an effective vaccine is not a simple step. There still remains the question as to the role of each T-cell population in the development of effective immunity (LIEW 1989) and that of how to selectively stimulate and generate long-term memory in the relevant subset of cells. Finally, the most appropriate vectors for inducing long-lasting protection are ill defined. Clearly, these are issues that must be resolved for individual microorganisms if effective modulation of the immune response is to be achieved.

References

Adorini L, Muller S, Cardinaux F, Lehmann PV, Facione R, Nagy Z (1988) In vivo competition between self peptides and foreign antigens in T cell cultivation. Nature 334: 623–625

Babbitt B, Allen P, Matsueda G, Haber E, Unanue ER (1985) Binding of immunogenic peptides to Ia histocompatibility molecules. Nature 317: 359–360

Bjorkman PJ, Saper MA, Samraoui B, Bennett WS, Strominger JL, Wiley DC (1987a) Structure of the human class I histocompatibility antigen, HLA-A2. Nature 329: 506–512

Bjorkman PJ, Saper MA, Samraoui B, Bennett WS, Strominger JL, Wiley DC (1987b) The foreign antigen combining site and T cell recognition regions of class I histocompatibility antigens. Nature 329: 512–518

Busch R, Howland K, Fenton C, Rothbard JB (1989) Binding of peptides to MHC class II proteins on B cell surfaces. Proc Natl Acad Sci USA (submitted)

Buus S, Sette A, Colon M, Jenis DM, Grey HM (1986) Isolation and characterisation of antigen-Ia complexes involved in T cell recognition. Cell 47: 1071–1075

Buus S, Sette A, Colon S, Miles C, Grey H (1987) The relationship between major histocompatibility complex (MHC) restriction and capacity of Ia to bind immunogenic peptides. Science 235: 1353–1358

Cease KB, Margalit H, Cornette JL, Putney SD, Robey WG, Onyang C, Streicher HZ, Fischinger PJ, Gallo RC, DeLisi C, Berzofsky JA (1987) Helpter T cell antigenic site identification in the AIDS virus gp 120 envelope protein and the induction of immunity in mice to the native protein using a 11-residue synthetic peptide. Proc Natl Acad Sci USA 84: 4249–4253

DeLisi C, Berzofsky JA (1985) T cell antigenic sites tend to be amphipathin structures. Proc Natl Acad Sci USA 82: 7048–7052

Gammon G, Shastri N, Cogswell J, Wilbur S, Sadegh-Nasseri S, Krzych N, Miller A, Sercarz E (1987) The choice of T cell epitopes utilised on a protein antigen depends on multiple factors distant from as well as at the determinant site. Immunol Rev 98: 53–75

Germain RN (1986) The ins and outs of antigen processing and presentation. Nature 322: 687–689

Good MF, Maloy WL, Lunde MN, Margalit H, Cornette JL, Smith GL, Moss B, Miller LH, Berzofsky JA (1987) Construction of synthetic immunogen: use of new T-helper epitope on malaria circumsporozoite. Science 235: 1059–1062

Howard M, Paul WE (1983) Regulation of B-cell growth and differentiation by soluble factors. Annu Rev Immunol 1: 307–334

Ivanyi J, Bothamley GH, Jackett PS (1988) Immunodiagnostic assays for tuberculosis and leprosy. Br Med Bull 44: 635–649

Kaufmann SHE (1988) $CD8^+$ T lymphocytes in intracellular microbial infections. Immunol Today 9: 168–174

Lamb JR, Ivanyi J, Rees ADM, Rothbard JB, Howland K, Young RA, Young DB (1986) Mapping of T cell epitopes using recombinant antigen and synthetic peptide. EMBO J : 1245–1249

Lamb JR, O'Hehir RE, Young DB (1988a) The use of nitrocellulose immunoblots for the analysis of antigen recognition by T lymphocytes. J Immunol Methods 110: 1–10

Lamb JR, Rees ADM, Bal V, Ikeda H, Wilkinson D, de Vries R, Rothbard JB (1988b) Prediction and identification of an HLA-DR restricted determinant in the 19kD protein of *Mycobacterium tuberculosis*. Eur J Immunol 18: 973–976

Liew FY (1989) Functional heterogeneity of $CD4^+$ T cells in leishmaniasis. Immunol Today 10: 40–45

Littman DR (1987) The structure of the CD4 and CD8 genes. Annu Rev Immunol 5: 561–584

Mehra V, Sweetser D, Young RA (1986) Efficient mapping of protein antigenic determinants. Proc Natl Acad Sci USA 83: 7013–7017

Moller G (ed) (1987) Antigen requirements for activation of MHC restricted responses. Immunol Rev 98: 1–187

Mossman TR, Coffman RL (1987) Two types of mouse helper T cell clone—implications for immune regulation. Immunol Today 8: 223–227

Mustafa AS, Gill HK, Nesland A, Britton WJ, Mehra V, Bloom BR, Young RA, Godal T (1986) Human T cell clones recognise a major *M. leprae* protein antigen expressed in *E. coli*. Nature 319: 63–66

Ottenhoff THM, Klatser PR, Ivanyi J, Elferink DG, de Wit MYL, de Vries RRP (1986) *Mycobacterium leprae* specific protein antigens defined by cloned human helper T cell clones. Nature 319: 66–68

Rothbard JB, Taylor WR (1988) A sequence pattern common to T cell epitopes. EMBO J 7: 93–100

Rothbard JB, Lechler RI, Howland K, Bal V, Eckels DD, Sekaly RP, Long EO, Taylor WR, Lamb JR (1988) Structural model of HLA-DR1 restriced T cell antigen recognition. Cell 52: 515–523

Rothbard JB, Busch R, Howland K, Bal V, Fenton C, Taylor WR, Lamb JR (1989) Structural analysis of a peptide-HLA class II complex: identification of critical interactions for its formation and recognition by T cell receptor. Int Immunol 1: 479–486

Shimonkevitz R, Kappler J, Marrack P, Grey H (1983) Antigen recognition by H-2 restricted T cell. I. Cell free antigen processing. J Exp Med 158: 303–316

Spouge JL, Guy HR, Cornette JL, Margalit H, Cease K, Berzofsky JA, DeLisi C (1987) Strong conformational propensities enhance T cell antigenticity. J Immunol 138: 204–212

Towbin H, Strachelin T, Gordon J (1979) Electrophoretic transfer of proteins from polyacrylamide gels to nitrocellulose sheets: procedures and some applications. Proc Natl Acad Sci USA 76: 4350–4354

Townsend ARM, McMichael AJ (1985) Specificity of cytotoxic T lymphocytes stimulated with influenza virus: studies in mice and human. Prog Allergy 36: 10–43

Townsend ARM, Bastin J, Gould K, Brownlee G, Andrew M, Coupar B, Boyle D, Chan S, Smith G (1988) Defective presentation to class I restricted cytotoxic T lymphocytes in vaccinia infected cells is overcome by enhanced degradation of antigen. J Exp Med 168: 1211–1224

Unanue ER (1984) Antigen presenting function of the macrophage. Annu Rev Immunol 2: 395–428

Watts T, Brian A, Kappler J, Marrack P, McConnell H (1985) Antigen presentation by supported planar membranes containing affinity purified $I\text{-}A^d$. Proc Natl Acad Sci USA 81: 7564–7568

Young DB, Lathigta R, Hendrix R, Sweetser D, Young RA (1988) Stress proteins are immune targets in leprosy and tuberculosis. Proc Natl Acad Sci USA 85: 4267–4270
YoungRA, Bloom BR, Grosskinsky CM, Ivanyi J, Thomas D, Davis RW (1985a) Dissection of *Mycobacterium tuberculosis* antigens using recombinant DNA. Proc Natl Acad Sci USA 82: 2583–2587
Young RA, Mehra V, Sweetser D, Buchanan T, Clark-Curtis J, Davis RW, Bloom BR (1985b) Genes for the major protein antigens of the leprosy parasite. Nature 316: 450–452

Development of BCG As a Recombinant Vaccine Vehicle*

W. R. JACOBS Jr., S. B. SNAPPER, L. LUGOSI, and B. R. BLOOM

1 Introduction

The bacille Calmette-Guérin (BCG) was developed by Dr A. Calmette and his associate Dr. C. Guérin at the Pasteur Institute in the early years of this century as a vaccine against tuberculosis. Despite enormous efforts by large numbers of experimental microbiologists of the time, the general methods for attenuating viruses and developing vaccines formulated by Pasteur had failed utterly on the tubercle bacillus. It was in this context that Calmette and Guérin, having difficulties in preventing clumping and aggregation of a virulent isolate of the bovine pathogen *Mycobacterium bovis* that they were studying, in 1906 decided to add ox bile to the culture medium to wet the surface of the organisms and disperse the cultures (CALMETTE and GUÉRIN 1909). The addition worked spectacularly, and the organisms grew almost as a single-cell suspension. In the course of 30 passages on bile, the colony morphology changed drastically, and the scientists realized that a profound genetic change might have been induced. Since the waxy coat of mycobacteria was believed to be critical to its resistance to killing by drying and to normal host defenses, they hoped that the change in morphology would be associated with a change in virulence. And so it was. As we now know, after many years of painstakingly detailed work in animals trying to select for variants or revertants to virulence, they were unable to do so and came to understand that they had developed an avirulent tubercle bacillus. In 1913 they showed that it could protect against lethal infection with virulent human *M. tuberculosis* in cows, guinea pigs, rabbits, and monkeys. After 231 passages, in July 1921, together with their colleague Prof. Weill-Halle, they inoculated their attenuated bovine bacillus, now immortalized by the name bacille Calmette-Guérin, into an infant "which was doomed to die of tuberculosis because it unavoidably lived with a consumptive grandmother—the mother, also consumptive, having died immediately after birth.

* This work was supported by grants from the UNDP/World Bank/WHO Special Programme for Research and Training in Tropical Diseases (IMMLEP and THELEP), the WHO Special Programme for Vaccine Development (IMMTUB), the United States Nationa Institutes of Health, and the Rockefeller Foundation

Department of Microbiology and Immunology, Albert Einstein College of Medicine, Bronx, NY 10461, USA

Current Topics in Microbiology and Immunology, Vol. 155

No incident ensued. The child has developed along normal lines and has since remained completely free of tuberculosis" (CALMETTE 1928).

Since that time, BCG vaccine remains the most widely used vaccine in the world (CALMETTE 1928). It has, since 1948, been used in billions of children all over the world and is included as one of the six childhood vaccines recommended for universal use in the Expanded Programme for Immunization of the World Health Organization. As a result of this program, the percentage of children immunized has risen from fewer than 20% in 1982 to 50% this year. Yet the effectiveness of BCG in controlling tuberculosis remains unclear and contentious. There are eight major controlled vaccine trials of BCG against tuberculosis (FINE 1985) and the efficacy has inexplicably varied enormously between trials. In the British MRC trial, BCG was 77% protective, but in the recent South Indian trial it engendered zero protection. Nevertheless, a reasonable interpretation of the data would hold that in almost all cases where it has been examined, BCG has protected against tuberculous meningitis and disseminated tuberculosis, and in some circumstances it can be effective in immunizing against pulmonary tuberculosis.

2 Recombinant BCG As a Multivalent Vaccine Vehicle

Despite the effectiveness of existing vaccines, each has some limitations that limit its usefulness. For example, while diphtheria-pertussis-tetanus vaccine is highly effective, the vaccine cannot be given until after maternal antibodies wane at 6–9 months, and it requires two booster shots to provide effective immunity, which in most developing countries is logistically difficult and expensive. There are many countries in which the experience is that 28% of the coverage is lost with each booster required. Therefore we recognize the urgent need for multivaccine vehicles or vectors that can provide effective immunity against multiple antigens, hopefully with a single immunization. We believe that a recombinant BCG polyvalent, along with recombinant vaccinia, salmonella, and adenoviruses, among others, have real potential to be developed into recombinant multivaccine vectors. The potential advantages may be summarized as follows:

1. BCG has been administered safely in over 2.5 billion doses since 1948, with a very low frequency of serious complications.
2. BCG is the only vaccine, other than oral polio, recommended by WHO to be given at birth.
3. BCG requires only a single immunization that can engender cell-mediated immunity to tuberculosis for 5–50 years.
4. BCG is the most effective known adjuvant for induction of cell-mediated immunity in animals and man.
5. BCG costs U.S. $0.55 per dose.

3 Development of Molecular Genetic Systems for Mycobacteria

Because BCG presents unique advantages for developing a recombinant polyvalent vaccine, despite the paucity of genetic and molecular information about mycobacteria, we embarked on a systematic molecular approach to develop a genetic system in mycobacteria that would permit genes encoding protective antigens from a variety of pathogens to be introduced and stably expressed in the BCG cell. At a minimum, the expression of recombinant DNA molecules into mycobacteria requires: (a) an efficient means of introducing foreign DNA into the mycobacterial cell: (b) recombinant DNA vectors that can replicate and be stably maintained in the mycobacterial host; and (c) expression of genes encoding selectable phenotypes for identifying cells containing recombinant DNA. Because of the slow generation time of BCG (24 h compared with 20 min for *Escherichia coli*), our initial studies were initiated with a fast-growing, non pathogenic mycobacterium, *M. smegmatis*. As illustrated in Fig. 1, there are two basic strategies for stably introducing the foreign DNA into bacterial cells: (a) integration of the foreign genes of interest into the mycobacterial chromosome by a phage-based recombination event or by homologous recombination, where they can be replicated as part of the chromosome, and (b) introduction of the foreign genes on an extrachromosomal, autonomously replicating vector, i.e., a plasmid. Because no mycobacterial plasmids containing selectable markers for mycobacteria existed, we initially screened a variety of plasmids useful in *Streptomyces* and *Bacillus* for their ability to transform *M. smegmatis*. To date, these attempts have failed totally.

To address the possibility that our failure was due to an inability of DNA to penetrate the cell wall and complex lipid coat of the cells, we developed methods for transfecting mycobacterial cells with mycobacteriophage DNAs. By adapting methods for producing spheroplasts, we were able to introduce phage DNA into mycobacterial cells with high efficiency (10^5 plaque-forming units per microgram of

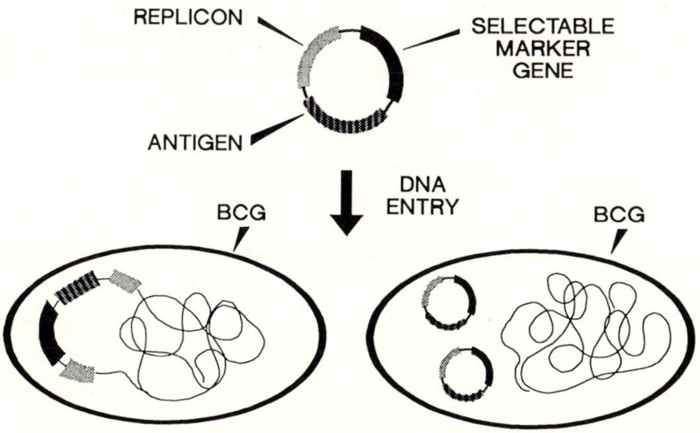

Fig. 1. General strategies for transformation of BCG. A useful vector must have a selectible marker, a replicon, and the gene of interest

phage DNA). When *Streptomyces* plasmids were introduced under the same conditions, transformation was still not achieved, indicating that the problem lay either in: (a) the inability to introduce "foreign" DNA molecules into mycobacterial hosts due to the degradation of "foreign" DNA by a host restriction system; (b) the lack of origin of replication that functioned in mycobacteria; (c) the failure to express the selectable marker gene in mycobacteria; or (d) our inability to reconstitute or regenerate bacterial cell walls from spheroplasts. Using mycobacteriophages as vectors, we were able to analyze and overcome these potential problems.

3.1 Phage-Based Strategy

Mycobacteriophages represent excellent candidates for recombinant DNA vectors for mycobacteria since many phages are known that infect and replicate in a wide range of both fast-growing and slow-growing mycobacterial species. To construct mycobacteriophage vectors, we exploited the observation that mycobacterial genes are not well expressed in *E. coli* (Jacobs et al. 1986a, b), thereby providing a state of conditional expression of mycobacteriophage DNA. We reasoned that we could clone into *E. coli* plasmids, fragments of mycobacteriophage DNA that would produce lytic phage if expressed in mycobacteria, and yet fragments that would not be expressed in *E. coli* and thus not lyse the *E. coli* cell. Borrowing the terminology from S. Brenner, we named such a construct a "shuttle phasmid," because it would replicate in mycobacteria as a phage and replicate in *E. coli* as a plasmid and be readily genetically manipulated. In addition, the strategy was to introduce recombinant phage DNA by transfection directly into a fast-growing *Mycobacterium*, such as *M. smegmatis*, following which the recombinant DNA molecules would then be packaged into mycobacteriophage particles. It then became possible to introduce the recombinant DNA in these phage particles by infection of slow-growing species of mycobacteria, such as BCG, at high efficiency. If mycobacteriophages that were temperate and nonlytic could be found, it should be possible then to introduce and stably express recombinant DNA in mycobacterial cells by lysogeny. We successfully utilized a cosmid cloning strategy and mycobacterial transfection to produce *E. coli*-mycobacteria shuttle phasmids, using the mycobacteriophage TM4 and the cosmid pHC79. These recombinant plasmids were shown to be capable of infecting both *M. smegmatis* and BCG vaccine substrains, thereby introducing recombinant DNA into both slow-growing and fast-growing mycobacteria for the first time (Jacobs et al. 1987). By comparing the transfection frequencies of shuttle phasmid DNAs isolated from *E. coli* or mycobacteriophage particles, we were able to show that *M. smegmatis* had no restriction system that recognized *E. coli* DNA as foreign, thus eliminating genetic restriction as the reason for unsuccessful transformation. Success was not altogether sweet, however, because the initial phage used, TM4, had been chosen because it had appeared to be a temperate phage isolated from *M. avium*. Although it may be capable of lysogenizing *M. avium*, we have been unable to date stably to lysogenize *M. smegmatis* or BCG with TM4 or TM4-derived shuttle phasmids. Consequently, we were obliged to start again from the beginning and screen a panel of mycobacteriophages to identify some that are truly temperate and stably lysogenize *M. smegmatis*. One such phage, L1, had been previously reported to be temperate. We confirmed the observations that it was capable of making *M. smegmatis* cells resistant to superinfection, as would be expected for a lysogen. In addition, we were able to demonstrate, by Southern analysis, that the L1 prophage integrates in a site-specific fashion into the *M. smegmatis* chromosome as its means of establishing lysogeny, the first such demonstration for a mycobacteriophage (SNAPPER et al. 1988). We were able to construct L1-shuttle phasmids in a manner analogous to the construction of TM4-shuttle phasmids and were gratified to observe that these phasmids retained the ability to lysogenize *M. smegmatis* (SNAPPER et al. 1988). We thus had, for the first time, the ability to introduce recombinant DNA into mycobacterial cells in a stable manner. Next we cloned into one such L1-shuttle phasmid a gene encoding kanamycin resistance and established that this gene conferred kanamycin-resistance to mycobacterial cells. This established the kanamycin-resistance gene and kanamycin as the first selectable marker gene system for the mycobacteria. Overall, these studies established lysogeny as one potentially useful means of introduce and express foreign genes in mycobacteria.

3.2 Plasmid-Based Strategy

Plasmid genetic system extend the capability of phages by offering increased cloning capacity, ease of DNA manipulation, and possibly increased copy number of the vector. Because of the lack of mycobacterial plasmids containing selectable markers, and our failure to transform mycobacteria using plasmids developed in other genera, a hybrid plasmid was constructed by T. KIESER and A. JEKKEL by ligating a full-length *E. coli* plasmid, pIJ666, containing a gene for kanamycin resistance, randomly into a cryptic mycobacterial plasmid, pAL5000, originally isolated from *M. fortuitum* (SNAPPER et al. 1988). When we transformed the library containing these inserts by electroporation into *M. smegmatis*, transformants resistant to kanamycin were found. Isolated plasmids from the transformants had the ability to replicate and transform both *E. coli* and mycobacteria. Further analysis of these transformants should indicate the mycobacterial plasmid DNA sequences required for replication (replicon). Of particular interest, conditions have now been developed, as well, for permitting transformation (10^4 transformants/μg DNA) by these hybrid plasmids of several BCG vaccine substrains at high efficiency, as illustrated in Fig. 2 (SNAPPER et al. 1988; LUGOSI et al. 1989).

4 Development of the Recombinant BCG Vehicle

Much remains to be done to develop BCG into a useful multivaccine vehicle. For constructing optimally effective vaccines, we will need to optimize the expression of the foreign antigens in BCG and define, in molecular terms, the important

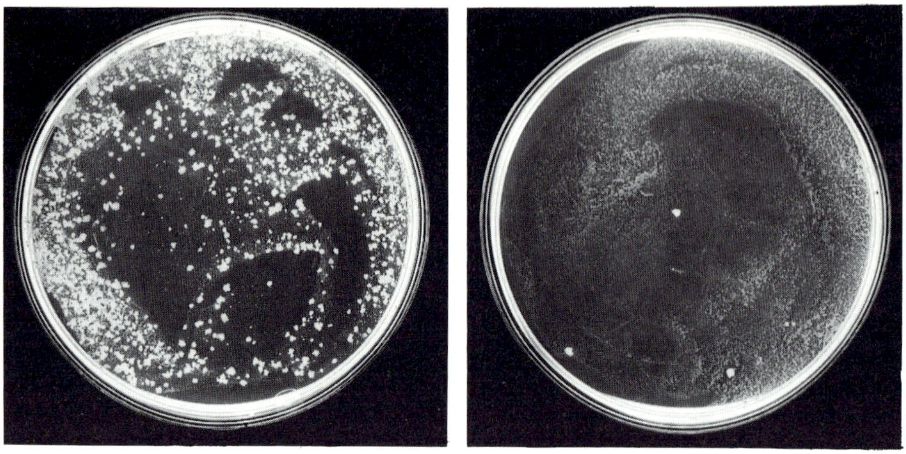

Fig. 2. Transformation of BCG with a recombinant shuttle plasmid, pYUB13, containing origins of replication for *E. coli* and mycobacteria. *Left*, the Pasteur BCG substrain transformed with shuttle plasmid containing the gene from Tn903 for kanamycin resistance and plated on medium containing kanamycin; *right*, mock transformed BCG plated on medium containing kanamycin

parameters for immunization of animals and humans. In order to achieve these goals, we will have to accumulate much additional basic knowledge of mycobacterial molecular biology and genetics.

4.1 Optimization of the Expression of Foreign Antigens

Ideally, we would like to express, in BCG, any open reading frame of DNA derived from any foreign antigen. The first necessity is to identify mycobacterial expression sequences. Mycobacteria contain high G-C DNA and, while related to gram-positive organisms, may have special DNA sequences useful for expressing foreign genes. We plan to use reporter genes, such as β-galactosidase, to identify mycobacterial promoters that will be used to transcribe genes encoding foreign antigens. These promoters will need to be characterized as to their efficiency of expression, and whether they are constitutive or regulated, to allow us to control expression of foreign genes. In addition, we will need to define and characterize the sequences necessary for efficient translation in the mycobacteria. Using this information, we should be able to construct a series of expression vectors that permit us to clone any open reading frame downstream from efficiently expressed transcriptional and translational elements. In addition, it may be necessary to develop regulated expression systems that will allow for expression of the foreign antigens in defined periods of growth of the BCG cell in the mammalian host in order to optimize the immune response.

Optimal expression of foreign antigens will require that the recombinant DNA constructs encoding the expressed foreign antigens are not lost during growth of the

BCG in the mammalian host. In order to ensure that these recombinant constructs are not lost, we will need to develop systems that select against the loss of the recombinant DNA. In general, antibiotic-resistant genes are inappropriate selectable markers for human vaccine vectors. We have begun to develop insertional mutagenic strategies that will allow us to isolate auxotrophic mutations in the BCG chromosome. A well-defined stable mutation and a complementing gene cloned on a plasmid offer alternative selection systems for stabilizing plasmid vectors. Such a system has been used successfully stably to maintain recombinant plasmids in *Salmonella* vaccine strains in vivo (NAKAYAMA et al. 1988.)

Alternatively, foreign genes could be placed in the BCG chromosome by using mycobacteriophage site-specific integration systems or homologous recombination systems of BCG. The advantage of this strategy is that the foreign genes are introduced into the host chromosome and may not require continuous selection; a disadvantage is that only a single copy can be introduced.

Optimal expression of foreign antigens in BCG will require that expressed protein be stably maintained in the BCG cell. It is clear that expression of some foreign genes in *E. coli* is limited by enzymes of the host capable of degrading foreign proteins selectively. It has been possible to stabilize expression by developing mutants in the host proteolytic enzymes in many instances in *E. coli* (GOLDBERG and ST JOHN 1976), and similar approaches may be useful to increasing stability of expression of foreign antigens in BCG.

4.2 Optimizing the Immunization Potential of Expressed Foreign Antigens: Targeting the Recombinant Antigens Produced To Be Secreted or Expressed in the Cell Wall

We have established that the major antigen(s) in *M. leprae* and *M. tuberculosis* recognized by T helper cells reside in the cell wall and that purified cell walls are immunogenic (MELANCON-KAPLAN et al. 1988). To increase immunogenicity, particularly for developing antibodies, and to prevent foreign proteins from becoming toxic to the BCG it may be advantageous to include mycobacterial signal sequences that will permit a significant portion of recombinant protein to be secreted from the recombinant BCG vector. An equally compelling immunological reason for developing recombinant BCG that can secrete introduced antigens derives from the elegant demonstration by BEVAN and associates (ROOTE et al. 1988) that in order to generate MHC class I restricted cytotoxic T lymphocytes it is obligatory for the antigen to be present in the cytoplasm of the antigen presenting and target cells. Targeting of recombinant antigens to the cell wall is attractive because of the high immunogenicity and adjuvanticity of mycobacterial cell walls. In addition, because of possible concerns with introducing a live vaccine in populations with a high prevalence of HIV seropositivity, nonliving, but highly immunogenic recombinant cell wall subunit vaccines provide a useful alternative to live vaccines. (It should be noted that there is little evidence at present that vaccination with BCG has increased the risk of untoward complications in such high-risk populations.) Overall, the recently developed genetic tools for studying and manipulating mycobacteria suggest that the limiting factor in development of recombinant BCG multivaccine vehicles will be biological problems, such as the nature of protective antigens and development of high levels of specific immune responses, e.g., antibodies or cytotoxic T cells, rather than genetic ones.

Acknowledgements. We are grateful for the outstanding assistance of Mrs. Margareta Tuckman, who contributed much to the experiments described, and to K. Ganjam, L. Pane and R. Barletta of our laboratory for very valuable discussion. We wish to thank Dr. Richard Young, Whitehead Institute and Dr. Ronald Davis of Stanford University for continuing helpful advice and criticism.

References

Brenner S, Cesaveni G, Karn Z (1982) Phasmids: hybrids between Co1E1 plasmids and *E. coli* bacteriophage lambda. Gene 17:27–44

Calmette A (1928) Preliminary statement on the method of preventive vaccination for tuberculosis with BCG. In: Report of the technical conference for the study of vaccination against tuberculosis by means of BCG. League of Nations Health Organization, Geneva, pp 22–47

Calmette A, Guérin C (1909) Sur qelques proprietés du bacilles tuberculeux d'origine bovine cultivé sur la bile de boeuf glycerinė Compt R Acad Sci 149: 716

Fine PEM, (1985) The role of BCG in the control of leprosy. Ethiop Med J 23: 179

Goldberg AL, St John AC (1976) Intracellular protein degradation in mammalian and bacterial cells. Annu Rev Biochem 45:747–803

Jacobs WR, Docherty MA, Curtiss R III, Clark-Curtiss JE (1986a) Expression of a *Mycobacterium* leprae genes from a *Streptococcus mutans* promoter in *Escherichia coli* K-12. Proc Natl Acad Sci USA 83:1926–1930

Jacobs W, Barrett RF, Clark-Curtiss JE and Curtiss R III (1986b) In vivo repackaging of recombinant cosmid molecules for analysis of *Salmonella typhimurium, Streptococcus mutans*, and mycobacterial genomic libraries. Infect Immun 52: 101–109

Jacobs WR Jr, Tuckman M, Bloom BR (1987) Introduction of foreign DNA into mycobacteria using a shuttle phasmid. Nature 327: 532–536

Lugosi L, Jacobs WR Jr, Bloom BR (1989) Genetic transformation of BCG. Tubercle (in press)

Melancon-Kaplan J, Wu Hunter S, McNeil M, Stewart C, Modlin RL, Rea T, Convit J, Salgame P, Mehra V, Bloom BR, Brennan PJ (1988) Immunological significance of *Mycobacterium leprae* cell walls. Proc Natl Acad Sci 85: 1917–1921

Moore MW Carbone FR, Bevan MJ (1988) Introduction of soluble into the class I pathway of antigen processing and presentation. Cell 54: 777–785

Nakayama K, Kelly SM, Curtiss R III (1988) Construction of an Asd^+ expression-cloning vector: stable maintenance and high level expression of cloned genes in a *Salmonella* vaccine vector strain. Biotechnology 6: 693–697

Snapper SB, Lugosi L, Jekkel A, Melton RE, Kieser T, Bloom BR, Jacobs WR Jr (1988) Lysogeny and transformation in mycobacteria: stable expression of foreign genes. Proc. Natl Acad Sci USA 85: 6987–6991

Subject Index